GOD'S Rx for HEALTH and WHOLENESS

JAMES P. GILLS, MD

SILOAM

Most Charisma House Book Group products are available at special quantity discounts for bulk purchase for sales promotions, premiums, fund-raising, and educational needs. For details, write Charisma House Book Group, 600 Rinehart Road, Lake Mary, Florida 32746, or telephone (407) 333-0600.

God's Rx for Health and Wholeness by James P. Gills, MD
Published by Siloam
Charisma Media/Charisma House Book Group
600 Rinehart Road, Lake Mary, Florida 32746
www.charismahouse.com

Visit the author's website at www.stlukeseye.com.

Library of Congress Cataloging-in-Publication Data:
An application to register this book for cataloging has been submitted to the Library of Congress.
ISBN: 978-1-62999-637-0
E-book ISBN: 978-1-62999-638-7

This book is not intended to provide medical advice or to take the place of medical advice and treatment from your personal physician. Readers are advised to consult their own doctors or other qualified health professionals regarding the treatment of their medical problems. Neither the publisher nor the author takes any responsibility for any possible consequences from any treatment, action, or application of medicine, supplement, herb, or preparation to any person reading or following the information in this book. If readers are taking prescription medications, they should consult with their physicians and not take themselves off of medicines to start supplementation without the proper supervision of a physician.

Portions of this book were previously published by Siloam as *God's Prescription for Healing*, ISBN 0-88419-947-9, copyright © 2004.

This publication is translated in Spanish under the title *La prescripción de Dios para la sanidad y la plenitud*, copyright © 2019 by James P. Gills, MD, published by Casa Creación, a Charisma Media company. All rights reserved.

19 20 21 22 23 — 987654321
Printed in the United States of America

CONTENTS

PREFACE

Great is the L*ORD, and greatly to be praised;*
and His greatness is unsearchable.
—PSALM 145:3

HAVE YOU SEEN mystery in a butterfly tenderly drying its wings under a ray of morning sunlight before it dances away on the breeze? Have you wondered at the language—or is it laughter—of dolphins? How often have you taken the time to enjoy, and appreciate, the spectacle of a full moon rising? Are you able to fully comprehend the ages, sizes, and distances of the galaxies of stars in an endless cosmos? And what can you make of the glorious chorus a songbird learns from its parents, or a pet dog's desire to please? All of created nature—the whole universe—points to the presence of an intelligence in its formation and function. However, nowhere is the thumbprint of a creator more visible than upon human life—upon your life.

In this book you will discover that the beginning and end of your healing—the truth of God's prescription—have been preplanned and designed. Healing was present before you were formed. This is the great, unsearchable miracle of life: all the wisdom that the Creator needs to create and preserve all humankind is already within you! In the design of intricate and delicate mechanisms—from molecular interactions to the teamwork of organs—the spiritually open eye willingly sees the evidence of the designer's plan for eternity with Him as well as life and healing now.

In its essence the message of the entire Bible is that mankind was created to enjoy divine rest. We were not created with a need just for physical rest but for divinely ordained rest that creates in us a harmony of spirit, soul, and body. This supernatural well-being for which God designed mankind is taught throughout the Old and New Testaments. It is available only to those who seek God, submit to His ways, and rest in His redemption. God spoke to His people of this provision for divine rest through the prophet Isaiah.

> This is the true rest [the way to true comfort and happiness] that you shall give to the weary, and, this is the [true] refreshing—yet they would not listen [to His teaching].
>
> —Isaiah 28:12, AMPC

You were made to live in intimate relationship with God the Father, God the Son, and God the Holy Spirit. Receiving the forgiveness available to every soul who comes to Christ in faith is the only true way to quiet the unrest of your humanity. The peace of God, which comes from accepting this forgiveness, will transform your heart and mind so that you can be restored to a life of resting in His redemption.

Perhaps we can better understand the concept of resting in His redemption through a story about my friend Jamie Buckingham. He had just been through a serious bout with cancer. He and I were walking on the beach, and I noticed he was quieter than usual. I assumed he was feeling poorly from the treatments and asked if he was OK. Jamie replied, "I've never been better. And my relationship with my wife is better than ever."

"But you've just been through a major health crisis. It would be perfectly normal to be struggling right now," I pointed out. "How can life be as good as you say?"

"Because I've come to the place where it's just Jamie and Jesus," he replied. "It's just Jamie and Jesus."

That is a picture of a believer who has surrendered his life totally to Christ and is resting in the redemption. When it's just you and God, the noisy distractions of life fade as your true priorities become crystal clear. You stop wasting time going through the motions and focus on what really matters. You live an authentic Christian life instead of playing the part of a Christian and keeping external rules. You become a true reflection of our Lord. As a result, you experience a peace you've never known before, and your heart earnestly echoes the words of hymnist Horatio Spafford: "It is well with my soul."

Unfortunately that has not been the daily experience of many Christians. They either have not understood or have not availed themselves of the true rest available to the believer in Christ. Making genuine relationship with God their first priority in life and entering into intimate communion with Him is a journey, but not all believers have made that journey the daily focus of their lives.

God's love is the starting point for our love and appreciation of others. It is the healing point. We have to receive His love before we are able to show appreciation to others and share His love with them. It is in His love that we can be restored to health and wholeness in every aspect of our lives.

If you desire to experience true health and wholeness, I invite you to open your heart and mind to God's amazing rest, peace, and joy, which are found in communion with Him. As you journey into the truth of the wondrous mystery of God's love for you, it may seem too good to be true. That is because the love of God is unlike anything this world has to offer. You will be ruined for any lesser, temporal pleasures or loves once you taste more deeply the divine wonder of resting in His redemption.

The facts of our creation are unimaginably profound. There is massive scientific proof of the infinite intelligence built physically into the zygote, determining the individual we each become. How can we not be living in awe, wonder, appreciation—and worship? Within our molecules are the record and testimony of a Creator's great care for every person born. This profound understanding of God's love for you is where God's Rx for health and wholeness resides.

—James P. Gills, MD

INTRODUCTION

A theory is the more impressive the greater the simplicity of its premises is, the more different kinds of things it relates, and the more extended its area of applicability.

—ALBERT EINSTEIN

THE INDESCRIBABLE COMPLEXITY in everything around us indicates an infinite, mysterious design for life. This complexity is found in the unbelievably immense and the unimaginably tiny. We can see it in distant star clusters, in the earth's weather patterns, in an elephant's memory, and in an ant's ability to find food. But nowhere is it more evident than the human body.

We have been created as *physical*, *mental*, and *spiritual* beings with a marvelous design. All of life, regarding sickness and healing, can be conceived in us as a reaction to injury that must be both appropriate and balanced. This is true for physical disease, mental trauma, or a lost and confused spirit. The grandeur of God's original design—His design for you—reveals His intent for health and wholeness, as seen on the cellular level, where every cell is assigned its particular task to that end.

When we cut a finger, for example, there is an immensely complex cellular response for repairing the area of the injury. Through an elaborate cascade of reactions, protein messages are sent and received. Vessels are narrowed accordingly, protective scabs are constructed, and cell duplication for the regeneration of new flesh begins. This all involves thousands and thousands of individual reactions among the trillions of atoms that make up the cells around the wound site. It is a process of unfathomable complexity, mystery, and mastery. And the same holds true for the body's reactions to tumors, herniated disks, broken bones, and cataracts. The bodies we inhabit for the duration of our brief lives on earth obviously contain impeccable wisdom and purpose.

More than in any other era, science has made this truth clear. Advances in biochemistry, molecular biology, and medicine have shown that the complexity of our own design is quite beyond complete comprehension and entirely beyond imitation. It is unconditionally beyond a detached process of the theory of evolution. It could only be derived from an intelligent source, from an intelligent designer. Intelligent design is revealed by science in the farthest planets as well as in intracellular detail. The observations of human science all point to the Designer, Creator, and Father. These visible proofs remind us of our need to appreciate Him. Sadly we are almost universally unobservant and ungrateful to Him for the wonder that is our creation.

THE NEED FOR UNDERSTANDING AND APPRECIATION

Many of us have a major fault within us: we take precious things for granted—the universe and living species on the planet as well as our bodies, our health, and our well-being—until we suffer their lack or loss. However, when we do lose something important, we become acutely aware of what we once had. It is then that we begin to look for answers—to try to make sense of the suffering we endure because of that loss of something precious in our lives. In those situations this profound principle emerges: we might never be awakened to the intelligence of the Creator in His creation unless we also experience some suffering in this life.

Brokenness, physical or otherwise, is not a simple condition that pills can cure—at least not often. You already know this if you are ailing. The emotions and reactions—the effects—that accompany suffering are as numerous as the possible illnesses themselves. This makes each person's experience, your experience, with illness unique.

We must learn to recognize the beauty of our design. We should be able to identify the intelligence in our design and be filled with wonder for our own existence. Why do we look without seeing and accept without cherishing? Even the normal function of our bodies should fill us with a sense of awe and appreciation for the intelligence behind it all. As we explore the miracle of our design—and question the meaning of our suffering—we will recognize the beauty of our creation and of the master designer behind it all.

When your body is suffering from the pain and limitation of illness, do you turn to your designer for His divine solutions? Or do you seek answers through a wide stream of competing natural influences and apparent answers? Maybe you turn to magazine articles or websites, for example. Or you lean toward the advice of friends or the attentions of doctors. Maybe you read whole texts on nutrition and exercise. Perhaps you have explored a large and growing number of available alternative (complementary) therapies and techniques for healing. Some of these alternatives are helpful, some are hopeless, and some are harmful.

It is in turning to your designer and His provision for your redemption and healing in Christ that you will receive true, divine guidance. That guidance is the necessary element to make appropriate decisions regarding your health. Your search for answers should start with seeking to know the Creator's intelligence, revealed in His loving care for you. As you seek to know Him through intimate relationship, He will lead you into the path of healing that is right for you. It is in prayer and communion with Him in your experience of illness that your pathway to healing will be made clear. Looking to the Lord for His guidance and seeking to understand His purpose for you will lead you to the health and wholeness that He wants for you. Through that humble seeking of God, many can be aided, uplifted, and healed.

Close scientific examination of the issues involved in your illness and deep spiritual contemplation in the Scriptures and in prayer will become the necessary medical and spiritual basis for your healing. You have been endowed with intellectual tools: human science and reason. Employing them, you may dive into the depths of the mystery of health and acquaint yourself, to some degree, with the Creator's plan.

And within that understanding—once you accept the truth of the sovereignty of the designer—you will discover insights into God's prescription for health and wholeness. Only by recognizing His divine design can you understand God's gifts and grace for your health and wholeness. Only then will you find within your heart the awe and true appreciation that are due our Creator.

Our scientific and spiritual understanding of healing, as well as our ability to effect healing in ourselves and in others, demands that we step back from our natural circumstances and observe the spiritual design of God for our entire well-being. We need to be ordinary people appreciating our extraordinary God.

PURPOSE

All things showing a *purity* of function also show a *purpose* of function that is directly due to a divine plan that was devised before their existence. You don't have to be a professional scientist to marvel at the endless beauty in nature and to see evidence of the plan for your health and wholeness. You only need to be willing to humbly acknowledge the intelligence of the Creator and be grateful for it. In that way you will come to understand your meaning and purpose.

Seeking God's wisdom to know your purpose will reveal His plan for your health and well-being as well. There are countless ways we may be ill, out of balance, and suffering. Likewise, there are numberless ways we may be healed—body, mind, and spirit. God's wisdom and mercy are unfathomable. By examining some key areas of our makeup in this book, we will take a look at God's provision of health and wholeness for the human body, mind, and spirit.

Meant to help you peer more deeply into the heart of God and His care of you, this book will be faith-reinforcing for those who believe in God's intent for their health and wholeness. It can also be a source of support for those who are suffering at present and need healing in their own lives. It can encourage those who desire to see healing in the lives of loved ones to know that God has designed the body for wholeness. He has also provided wisdom to physicians to be able to restore wholeness and health. This book may also become a reinforcement of that fact in the lives of sincere believers who distrust medical science, thinking that prayer alone is the pathway to healing.

Your health and wholeness have been designed, engineered, and given substance through God's amazing design in creation. Whatever your situation at present, my prayer is that you may be encouraged as we discuss these and other issues regarding God's wonderful, loving plan for your health and wholeness. All of His knowledge and provisions for the restoration of your health are coded into your body. Are you ready to tap into that knowledge? Let's begin.

CHAPTER 1

DIVINE DESIGN **IN CREATION**

THE INTELLIGENCE AND intentions of a divine designer have wholly unique expressions in every kind of creature on the planet. It is an intelligence constructed into the angles of bodies and the aptitudes of brains. It begins with a molecular intelligence that makes the requirements of life as an aardvark possible for the aardvark, which are very different from the requirements of life for the accountant. This divine intelligence is ratcheted into all the individual cells that originate from a single one. It is an intelligence that oversees and conducts the most colossal, perplexing, and rousing chorus of creativity in existence. That ultimate symphony is the breathing, heaving, extravagant economy of life on this planet.

The more carefully we look into the scientific discovery of these molecular processes of life, the more directly we are introduced to the infinite sophistication of a design that is responsible for all things. The science of our present age is finally exposing this phenomenon of the intricate design of life. Significant details are evident to the eye of the scientist at the cellular level in dimensions of nanometers (billionths of a meter).

Still, while mysteries of nature such as the Milky Way,

whale sonar, or the improbable flight of bumblebees can captivate our attention, in this text we want to concern ourselves as human beings with the basis of our own nature and our place in the universe. So, turning to the human body, we find the most astonishing proof of ingenuity, wisdom, and complexity woven into its natural design. And we see that proof most clearly in the genetic code of the single, all-generating zygote.

For generations, prevailing scientific theories have chosen to describe the phenomenon of life as the product of frigid physical forces and biochemical accident. Any competing concept of direction and design in nature has been ridiculed as superstition by these scientists who embrace theories of evolution. However, because of the recent profound scientific discoveries, a concept of design and an expression of deep wisdom controlling that design can now be understood to be a *scientific principle.* Within a single cell is the revelation of that truth that underlies all nature—including you and me. The human body represents a scientific revelation of the presence and personality of an intelligent designer of great wisdom who loves and heals.

You were designed—you are not a chemical accident—and that means you are full of meaning and purpose in the mind of the designer. Within this meaning and purpose are all the reasons to be alive and to stay alive. The designer has a plan for you that includes awesome mechanisms for maintenance of your well-being. The design of the human body provides countless powerful means to respond to injury and disease. The provisions for proper, precise, and efficient operation within you, and in each individual, expose the design and the prescription for health and wholeness.

Through an exploration of disease and the design for its healing you can find the hand of the designer at work. Through that discovery you will be able to understand the purpose and meaning of your structure and, more importantly, your meaning and purpose in life. And so not only is it *useful* to recognize and understand the natural design of your body to promote your health and healing, but it is a personal responsibility you must accept.

As each of us recognizes and embraces that responsibility, we can learn to gratefully acknowledge our health as our greatest earthly wealth. Nothing could be dearer. Also, in that acknowledgment we may look for the glorious face of the Creator in full appreciation of this, His gift to us.

DISCUSSION QUESTIONS

List the ways you find evidence of the intelligence and intentions of a divine designer in nature.

What physical aspects of your own body reveal God's intelligent design to you?

Read Proverbs 30:24–28 and explain how a scripture such as this one about God's tender care of and attention to His creation gives you hope for complete wholeness in your body.

CHAPTER 2

THE BASICS OF **DISEASE AND HEALING**

If you are looking for healing, for freedom from pain or disability—as each of us does through the course of life—it can be difficult to understand completely what is happening to you or why. Common terms regarding sickness are sometimes confusing, so it will be helpful to briefly distinguish a couple of important concepts at the start. Let me explain how the terms *disease* and *illness* relate to each other and how both relate to healing.

When you become sick, your body becomes an impediment to rather than an instrument of your purpose. In a state of illness your entire experience of existence becomes altered in a negative way. Those who become ill "experience a series of intimate insults to those aspects of their existence that are most integral to being human."[1] That is, when we are ill, we have lost the capacity for living in the manner to which we have grown accustomed.

A disease is a physical condition characterized by diminished or inappropriate function in the body. It is an imbalance in biological systems or structures. *Illness*, on the other hand, is all the uncomfortable and disturbing mental conditions and emotions that a person struggles with when *disease* is present in the body. Human illness, then, is illness of the whole person—body, mind, and soul—often caused by disease.

Curing illness has to do with eradicating disease. *Healing* has to do with restoring the whole person from the effects of illness.[2] We can only accomplish such complete restoration to health and wholeness through mental and spiritual adjustments, as well as eradicating the physical effects of the disease. Stated another way, authentic healing requires the physical cure as well as the restoration of mental and spiritual wholeness. We will refer to that blissful state as *total health.*

THE BASICS

The primary characteristic of both cure and healing, more than anything else, is described by the term *balance.* The human body—your body—was designed to maintain balance and make necessary adjustments when that natural balance is overturned. Take the relatively simple examples of the effect of heat and cold on your body. When you become chilled, you start to shiver. By this mechanism your body is trying to generate heat and reestablish balance of the appropriate body temperature. Likewise, when the environment is hot, your body's temperature is raised and the body restores balance through the mechanism of sweating. The evaporation of sweat off the skin is intended to bring rebalance, to lower the temperature in the body to its preferred level.

In this chapter we will focus on disease and cure for the physical body, which the designer coded into the body's innate healing abilities. How did He design our bodies to provide balance maintenance? When we speak about innate biological mechanisms, a scientific, empirical approach to the body as a grouping of organs and systems is most helpful.

Diseases can approach the body from the outside in the form of microorganisms, such as viruses, bacteria, and parasites. Trauma or disease may result from accidents, abuse, or exposure to chemicals and other harmful substances. Some diseases, such as cancer, originate within the body. In that particular case something has tipped the balance of the innate mechanism that normally checks errant cell growth within the body.

If we define the basis of all disease as a response to injury, then the basis of the cure of disease is the appropriate—balanced—physical response by the body's inborn mechanisms. The body has many, many such mechanisms that exist simply to respond to upset in the normal balance of function. Some of these still remain beyond our ability to explain. However, even the most unremarkable event of self-cure can be interpreted as a fantastic performance of coordinated and perfectly appropriate responses to injury.

Each tissue in the body displays an almost inexplicable complexity in its rejuvenating and renewing capacities. And this is observed in even the most mundane (least urgent) examples of its response to disease and illness. We are wholly mistaken when we take these for granted. Even this innate healing mechanism for a simple paper cut is a demonstration of our body's finely tuned sentry and repair systems. These functions derive directly from nature's fabulous design, all contained, initially, in the zygote.

Though each human body is unique, each is also the same, built upon the same model of design and balance initiated by a common wisdom and intelligence. When you think about the intelligence of another individual, or of yourself, you are thinking about that person's mental ability to problem-solve and to manipulate abstractions. Concerning the body, though, you must understand that the whole body exhibits an innate intelligence. Your immune system, for example, has a memory and "learns." You experience well-being to the extent that you do because your body is continually monitoring, laboring, regrowing, and fighting threatening elements intelligently.

How is it all accomplished? Why is it all accomplished? Most theorists would try to have you believe that such wondrous abilities and capacities of our physical bodies merely evolved from a great universal emptiness—from nothing. However, current cellular study provides evidence, at the molecular level, that the human body is the most lavish, intricate, and misunderstood piece of engineering in the universe.

Many students of science, like me, have had to embrace the truth revealed under the microscope of the exquisite beauty and complexity of design we see there. And many of us have been willing to acknowledge the designer Himself as God, who has become our Lord and Master. He has won our hearts, not only by the wonders of creation we have observed but by His infinite love revealed to us.

When we come to God through Christ, our Savior, His purpose for which we were created begins to fill our hearts and minds with joy and peace in discovering our eternal significance. Since that discovery I have been involved in a journey into the heart of God, learning to know Him through the Scriptures and in communion with Him in prayer and fellowship with other believers. I am continually seeking to rest more fully in His redemption in all of life's situations. And as I do, I find a place of deeper worship of my Savior. His love for me has given me a great desire to help others know the purpose for which they were born and to help them be restored to health and wholeness—body, mind, and spirit.

DISCUSSION QUESTIONS

List any illnesses or diseases you've been dealing with.

What physical symptoms are you experiencing that might be connected to these diseases?

What is the first step you will take toward your healing?

Write a scripture that gives you hope.

CHAPTER 3

DESIGNED FOR HEALTH AND WHOLENESS

NO PHYSICAL SYSTEM in the body functions perfectly. The immune system, the cornea, and the skin all have their points of occasional weakness. Yet even in our world filled with contaminants in air, water, and food, look at what they do accomplish for you! The odds are stacked against us biologically in a world so full of danger: mutating SARS viruses in the air, salmonella in our chicken, E. coli in our hamburger, and West Nile virus in the mosquitoes buzzing by our ears. These are a mere handful of familiar threats posed to our physical bodies.

Yet with scientific acuity we must observe the massive accomplishments of the intricate, sophisticated systems that we "own" from the moment we begin to develop as a person from a minuscule zygote. In the face of an impossibly huge number of threats, we mostly continue to survive. This survival and hope for healthiness would be meaningless if it were not for the Creator's intelligence, which is expressed in defense mechanisms throughout the entire body. There is undoubtedly an irreducible complexity built into us that is still beyond our ability to understand. That beautiful complexity asks each one of us to acknowledge and worship its Creator, our Creator, in deep appreciation and in awe and wonder of such profound beauty.

Ravi Zacharias has considered the heart of wonder and the dynamic of wonder in the heart, which he recorded in his book *Recapture the Wonder.* He wrote that you may think of wonder as "childlikeness in its sublimity."[1] It is right to think so. Wonder is the emotional experience that causes our eyes to widen and our hearts to race with excitement. The dream of ultimate fulfillment, the conscious and unconscious pursuit of life, is in wonder—in the balance of enchantment with reality.

For some, the more personal knowledge of stars and atoms and T cells they attain, it seems, the less wonder they seem to enjoy. This should not, nor need not, be the case. In fact knowledge of our human bodies and their many mechanisms and systems for life and health ought to excite and enhance our curiosity and wonder to no end! Deep mysteries in nature, our nature, can only prompt awe and wonder for the intelligence, the Creator, Father, who designed all and understands everything. It is because He understands everything that He has given us the searching minds we have. Human science provides us with a tiny taste of the deep design and loving care built into the zygote's DNA and the body that it generates. That is a design so unbelievably remarkable, awe-inspiring, mysterious, and wonderful that we must—really must—be grateful to God every moment that we are breathing.

Even so, the evidence exposed by modern scientific method continues to be largely interpreted by most within the terms of Darwinism and the theory of evolution. That does not add up. Interpreted honestly and humbly, details of our nature actually point to an *irreducible complexity*—that is, the scientific principle that describes an entity that could not be the product of mindless, directionless natural selection.

What science does tell us, if we are humble enough to believe it, is that within our organs, tissues, cells, DNA code, and subcellular molecular particles is the source for immense wonder. And it is—or should be—our main inspiration for great appreciation for our Creator. In the organization of our atoms, proteins, and integrated systems is the evidence that we were created with a marvelous, miraculous design intended not only to define but also to promote and prolong our physical existence on the earth according to a divine plan.

In the present era the existence of an everlasting soul and the dignity of each one of us—unique and precious in God's sight—have been denied by many. However, actual scientific facts observable in a solitary fertilized egg give us a startling account of the beautiful mind of the Creator. The natural defenses and responses of the human body also give us a clear expression of God's love and His plan for, and method of, our healing. God hands us His calling card through the scientific facts of our ability to exist, to flourish, and to heal when stricken.

This innate ability of the body to heal itself is God's first gift of healing. As recipients of this marvelous gift of creation, why do we not see this and love the Creator for it? Why are we not filled with appreciation? We cannot look at the body, at the amazing zygote, without seeing the face of God. Looking at the marvels of creation, we may rekindle the wonder in our hearts through a spirit of deep appreciation and gratitude for the gift.

Without doubt within our structure is the design for healing; however, we are a mortal creation, and the human body is fallible. The fact that we need healing at all means that we, our bodies, have the potential to falter and fail. In the occasional imbalances of the body, we come to see that sickness is as much a part of life as health is. Restoration is the goal we reach for, and it still may sometimes be outside the reach of natural systems alone. In such cases we must look outside of ourselves for some assistance. That is the idea, truth, and divine gift that we want to consider next.

DISCUSSION QUESTIONS

Have you tried to restore your health through your own research and wise choices? What were the results?

Have you sought the help of a doctor to deal with your illness?

What is the difference between treating an illness and preventing one?

CHAPTER 4

THE ROLE OF PHYSICIANS IN GOD'S Rx

TRY NOT TO despair—ever. A great intelligence has gone before you and anticipated your needs. You have been designed for healing. We have seen that the human body—your very own body—is wonderful and mysterious in the complexity of that design. It is a magnificent testimony to the Creator's design of the universe. With its ability to operate and maintain itself, the human body is the highlight of all created nature.

Yet it is true we are mortal. We must understand that as organic beings we are caught in continuous biological battles for strength, health, and existence. Deadly microorganisms, injuries, neuromuscular diseases, and daily stress are a few dangerous possibilities among an almost infinite number of other threats to our health.

Our vulnerability to so many varied attacks makes it a certainty that the human body will lose some of those battles. However, some of the resulting breakdowns in physical systems need not lead to permanent impairment, pain, or death, as we usually fear. Interruptions in proper function can be influenced and even reversed when true understanding of and appreciation of the body's systems are applied to their care, cure, and methods of prevention.

Often the difference between health and illness or life and death lies in the skillful, informed application of medical knowledge to the situation at hand. That is knowledge that begins with the understanding of the miracle of innate systems of healing contained in the cells that originate from the zygote. In other words, the road to well-being sometimes lies in finding assistance for the natural processes of healing our bodies possess. Our collective knowledge of the intricate human design provides helpful instruction for our judicious intervention.

Illness is a common human experience. Even the healthiest individuals among us cannot completely escape it. Still, it may not be easy for a person to admit to the need for assistance when his or her natural healing mechanisms have become injured, inadequate, or overtaxed. However, an authentic appreciation of the miracle of the body will raise awareness of and concern for the maintenance of its balance. When you are able to view life as the gift that it is, you will become committed to taking diligent care of it, just as you would tend a garden. You will desire to do whatever you can to remain healthy and to flourish. Taking care of your body is an important responsibility. That responsibility encompasses pursuing the wisdom and methods of healing provided by the collective human knowledge of the single cell and your wonderful design.

To be healed—to fulfill the meaning of your design for healing—sometimes you will need to change the food that you eat, sometimes you will need to find a bandage, and sometimes you will need to see a doctor. Always you would be judicious to present your need for healing in prayer to your loving God and Father. He will give you His peace and lead you to the pathway of healing that you need in your situation.

MEDICAL SCIENCE, THE PHYSICIAN, AND HEALING

The essence of medical science is the observation of, appreciation of, and careful intervention in the natural design of a person when it is needed to bring healing. In medicine our practice is bound as tightly to our scientific understanding of the manifestations of the Creator's knowledge as fruit is to the tree. In our age knowledge of the structures and functions of a body derived from a zygote is the base of the tree that bears the fruit of the physician's methods of healing.

When you are sick or injured, you turn for healing to those men and women who must do their jobs within their understanding of our created design. They examine, interpret tests, administer medication, and repair or alter with surgery. You anticipate their knowledge and skill to bring you comfort and relief—and to restore you. They employ techniques and apply scientific knowledge to reestablish the integrity of a body whose natural ability to defend or develop is enfeebled, broken down, or nonexistent. They apply the techniques in line with principles of nature, of the divine design of the body.

I have had personal experience with this creative use of healing techniques as a patient rather than a physician. After a bicycle accident during training years ago I suffered a severe and painful break in the femur, the large upper bone, of one leg. Dr. Dean Cole restored my leg with a vision of universal principles—physics, columns, load-bearing—along with an intimate understanding of human bones and their growth. He introduced an invention of his own into my broken leg, which allowed the damaged bone to lengthen from the inside as it healed. Over the period of a few months the bone grew a necessary two and one-half inches, which it would not have done through traditional treatment.

Profound understanding of the mechanics of the body's design and function within universal laws is what God has provided humanity as a result of scientific knowledge gained through centuries of observation of the human anatomy. Doctors must use this understanding in their efforts to heal. Therefore, your accepting responsibility for your body in illness often leads you to the doors of physicians in your hour of need. As stewards of our bodies, which the Scriptures describe as God's temples (1 Cor. 6:19–20), we must seek the knowledge and expertise of those who are familiar with the design. Those people are our physicians, and we should be willing to accept their assistance in our healing.

The following examples will help demonstrate the role of physicians and medical scientists in assisting in our healing.

GENETIC ENGINEERING

Not all cures of diseases are accomplished by medical practitioners alone. Medical researchers have an equally vital role to play. One exciting example of the human drive toward effecting cure within the boundaries of natural design is the cutting-edge research in genetic engineering. Through genetic engineering, formally known as recombinant DNA technology, medical science has been working with the DNA of humans and other species of life to attempt to cure certain diseases.

The process is elegant, at least in principle: scientists can remove genes from one organism and combine them with genes in a second organism. This allows the second organism to produce proteins, which the first organism does naturally but the second does not. The second, implanted organism gains the ability—through this introduced piece of DNA—to produce the proteins that the first organism naturally produces. Certain important substances can thus be produced in higher volumes this way.

Another aspect of recombinant DNA technology is replacing defective or missing genes with normal genes. Studies have found that there are many possible solutions to serious medical problems with the use of recombinant DNA gene therapy. Cancer treatment is only one. Others include help for patients who have inoperable heart disease. Such gene therapy has the potential to "become a major advancement in the treatment of heart disease."[1]

You may be aware that the human genome—the whole map of human genes—has been laid out in its entirety. DNA is mind-boggling in its complexity, and it is still not fully understood. The human DNA base pair sequence is one hundred times the number of strings of single-letter characters in an eighteen-volume *World Book Encyclopedia* set. That's three billion base pair sequences. Each of us differs by about one million pairs. The successful genome project mapped the DNA of only one individual, however.

This incredible scientific knowledge should create a profound awe and deep respect for created nature and our physical construction. It should humble us before God to worship Him for His greatness and His love for all of creation, especially mankind, whom He made in His image. (See Genesis 3.) We won't always be able to improve on nature. Yet such humility and appreciation for God's love for us will allow us to continue to forge new therapies for a body that was created so magnificently.

UNDERSTANDING DISEASE VS. ILLNESS

The medical and surgical interventions of physicians, as well as the efforts of researchers, do not describe the full efforts pursued in the role of physician-assisted healing. It is necessary to remember that when we are speaking of healing, we are referencing the need of people. The burden, and privilege, of all of us who seek to assist the healing of others is to address the humanness of those in need.

For example, it may be human nature that we are not focused in our recognition and appreciation of the good that we have in life but are all too aware of the bad. This negative perspective of life affects our thinking regarding sickness and health as well. In fact as unconscious of our blessings as we tend to be, we will sometimes think of health only as an absence of pain or disability. In other words, health is merely a lack of hindrance to our physical lives.

People with that limited perspective of health do not wake up in the morning thankful for the smooth-running efficiency of their bodies. Yet they are abruptly thrust into consciousness of their health when sickness strikes their bodies and becomes an obstruction to what they have taken for granted as health. Simple, daily functions—thinking, speaking, eating, or walking—once not part of their conscious thoughts become a paramount focus when these people are affected by injury or sickness. When they are faced with disease or illness, they will need to apply a proper understanding of what these terms involve in order to be restored to wholeness and health.

A proper understanding of healing, health, and wholeness pivots on the understanding of the meaning of *illness* as distinguished from the meaning of *disease*. Remember, *disease* is a process that causes biological malfunction; *illness* is the lived experience in the psyche and emotions and painful limitations caused by this biological malfunction. Illness involves a whole range of an individual's feelings and moods—fear, helplessness, powerlessness, dependency, and vulnerability. Disease, rather, is a neutral, objective, and scientific description of dysfunction in the biology of the body.[2] Both words might simply seem to connote a single state defined by its being a state of *unhealth*. However, even a minor sickness could conceivably cause a person a confrontation with his or her mortality. For that reason illness cannot be taken as a simple lack of health or the isolated experiences of pain and limitation caused by disease. It is a state of being that affects the life of the whole person.

For example, the experience of illness will be very difficult for an Olympic runner who is told that after her injury heals, she will be able to walk normally but will never run competitively again. Clearly this is one personal world instantly turned upside down, affecting her psyche and emotional well-being and requiring a changing of her goals in life.

For another individual who suffers the same injury as the Olympic runner but to whom creating art is the important achievement of life, the same bad news is not so difficult to receive. For these two people, whose injuries and physical pain are equivalent, the experience—the illness—has vastly different effects on their psyches and emotional well-being, as well as their futures.

Think also of the person who feels something is amiss in his or her physical health and becomes fearful, choked with anxiety. When the doctor can find no physical malfunction, we may think of this person as suffering an illness—fear and anxiety—without an actual disease affecting his or her health. Likewise, disease without illness can manifest itself in an individual who has had a physical weakness identified by a doctor yet feels good, remains irrepressibly positive, and refuses to see herself as sick.[3]

For health and wholeness to be restored, a person will need to embrace changes in his or her perspective of and goals for life. Those changes may involve the person's physical pursuits, mental perspective, and spiritual being.

MEDICAL CURE VS. TOTAL HEALING

"Disease is a territory colonized by science, with death lurking in the background, lining the horizon. And between these experiential extremes—that of the mortal self, and that of the neutral eye of science—innumerable [healing techniques] of experience are dispersed."[4] Doctors employ scientific knowledge to reestablish the integrity of a body. Yet can you say that this describes all that they do or all that you might hope for as a patient? Is this the path to or meaning of health and wholeness? Your answers lie in the way you understand humanity and what it means to be sick, and in your acknowledgment that the Creator remains the source of all health and wholeness—even through His instruments: your doctor's head and hands.

How is *health and wholeness* best defined under the requirements of cure and caring, with death lurking in the background?

Primarily the presence of both illness and disease requires a dialogue between patient and doctor that covers a wide range of potential physical and emotional experiences. *Cure* can proceed in a one-dimensional approach—advancing scientific techniques have allowed doctors to cure disease without a more intimate sense of care. But *healing* may not become a reality for the person if, after the removal of pain, limitation, and threat of death from that disease, fear and a sense of loss remain.

The personal and subjective nature of health and illness represent the need for balance in each life. When a development—a lump or pain or weakness—becomes alarming enough, that balance is shaken; you seek professional help. At this point you become a patient. Your doctor's treatment is a response to the partial disintegration of your being and constitutes the need for caring restoration of your individual balance of health and wholeness in your psyche as well as your body. There are several main elements that should characterize physicians' treatments who seek to care as well as cure. This brief explanation of the role of physicians in your healing provides some of the understanding you need as you seek their professional assistance to restore yourself to health and wholeness.

Understanding and respect

The human body is a natural wonder with an almost impenetrable biological design. The cure of disease is the realm of medicine that requires a scientific approach to the atoms, enzymes, receptors, organs, and systems of the body. This informs a technologically based repair and rejuvenation of impaired function and renewal of the integrity of the biological organism. There should be an element of awe, humility, and respect in the physician for the sheer magnificence of design and function in the human body, for its tissues, and every component part, down to its individual cells and molecules.

When that element of respect is present in the physician's treatments, the patient will be more hopeful and feel a sense of dignity as God's highest creation. They may more readily look to God for spiritual help and trust in their relationship with Him and His love for them, which brings rest and healing to their minds and spirits.

Knowledge and competence

The reason you visit an ophthalmologist rather than a gardener when you have trouble with your eyes is to benefit from the specific knowledge and training that the eye doctor possesses to apply to your difficulty. If health of the individual is the aim of the practice of medicine, this will mean that biomedical science and technology must be brought to bear on the problem. With a view of the patient as a fellow human, as a unique and precious creation of God, the physician has the obligation to provide craftsmanship and fully developed skills. All procedures must be carried out with attention to detail and perfection.

Compassion

We typically, and justifiably, think of *medicine* as a science, but our discussion of illness indicates that the practice of medicine is a *human* science—that is, the whole person is submitting to the physician's expertise to bring wholeness and health to him or her. Likely this is what people intuitively understand as the *art* of medicine. Illness and suffering cannot be treated without an understanding of people and the commensurate empathy for them. All doctors naturally depend upon biomedical experience and insights but also know too well that the same treatment can succeed in one patient and fail in another. The physician, to truly heal, must comprehend the patient's pain and suffering mentally and emotionally and recognize the patient as a fellow human who is "just like me." This will inevitably allow responsiveness to the unique aspects and needs of the patient.

Dignity of personal assistance

This element of healing is perhaps associated more with the services of nurses—as well as family members and friends—than of doctors. It entails doing for others what they cannot do for themselves. It is the provision of assistance in acts of living, such as cooking, feeding, bathing, and providing humor and emotional support. Guarding the dignity of the person who is needing assistance of another for things he or she is comfortable doing for himself or herself is vital to the healing process.

Offering assurance to the patient

The physician must be aware of several things in inviting the patient to trust and to transfer responsibility and anxiety. First, for the patient the relationship can seem unequal and cause the patient to feel insecure. The patient lacks the knowledge and means to effect his or her own cure and must supplicate others—usually strangers—for their help. This entails relinquishing a degree of freedom of choice and autonomy. Naturally feelings of vulnerability and lost dignity abide in the essence of this relationship. Self-image is as much at stake as biological health.

THE PHYSICIAN'S ROLE IN HEALING

> But a certain Samaritan, as he journeyed, came where he was. And when he saw him, he had compassion. So he went to him and bandaged his wounds, pouring on oil and wine; and he set him on his own animal, brought him to an inn, and took care of him.
>
> —Luke 10:33–34

Physician-assisted healing will be most effective when it expresses the love of Christ—*agape* love—as in Jesus' story of the charitable Samaritan. A philosophical or naturalistic ethic of doing perceived good to a patient is not sufficient. The Hippocratic Oath is a nonbinding declaration that is largely irrelevant in an age of unbridled technological advances. Confused ethics seek to guide us into the intractable debates surrounding, for example, cloning and abortion.

Medicine in its essence is a scientific pursuit with its own logic in *scientific* goals. But the broader sense of charitable treatment of a patient involves fidelity to the goal of the well-being of the patient; that becomes medicine's moral obligation and goal. This moral obligation can only be fulfilled by a physician who has surrendered his life to the love of Christ and desires to minister to patients out of that reservoir of divine love he or she has received.

Jesus gave us the purest example of the way Christian physicians should approach the sick. Healing those who were sick and suffering was a daily aspect of His life. Healing the ill was central to His mission to save. Faith, hope, integrity, and respect for the patient are elements that grow out of *agape* love—that is, the love that emanates from God Himself. It is the compassion, inspired by the example of our great physician, that enables health care professionals to recognize that, effective as our science and technology may be, they do not remove suffering. It is only the healing love of Christ shared with a patient that can go deeper than physical pain and relieve the suffering of the psyche and spirit of a man or woman. This spiritual reality makes the pursuit of Christian physicians to know God in an intimate relationship a more profound necessity to their ultimate success.

In reality physicians are meant to be God's instruments to apply healing principles and techniques for cure that God has provided. Through the knowledge and wisdom they have discovered in their study of medical science, compiled over centuries, physicians can seek the wisdom of God for the healing of each patient.

When you become a patient, prayerfully seek the guidance of God to submit yourself to the skillful hands of trained physicians, those who not only employ technological advances to your situation but seek to know God's wisdom for your healing. In that way you can expect God to be with you and to teach you to rest in His love for you as you see restoration of health and wholeness.

DISCUSSION QUESTIONS

Did you start your search for your health answers by consulting God and His Word? Or did you rely on human efforts to seek a cure?

Does your doctor incorporate elements of care in his or her treatment, or does he or she only focus on the cure?

Have you ever had to seek a second opinion when it comes to your medical care? What was the outcome?

CHAPTER 5

YOUR PERSONAL ROLE IN GOD'S Rx

NOTHING CAN REPLACE the expertise of physicians in our lives, and you should not hesitate to seek their help when it is required. To fail to do that would be to deny one of the great gifts God has provided for your health and wholeness. When you feel out of control in a time of sickness, you want someone to take control who understands your situation. That makes good sense. The complexity of the body, its diseases, and the gap in knowledge of those issues has most of us at a loss as to what to do. Also, we have fears of the unknown world of sickness and its potential consequences. The Creator loves you and has given physicians knowledge and understanding of the cause of and cure for your physical or psychological pain.

However, you have a responsibility to take an active role in your healing process as well. A doctor can treat a disease, or at least its symptoms. But it will be harder for the patient to heal if the patient doesn't recognize his or her own responsibility and take an active role in the healing process. A return to wholeness requires substantially more than receiving a medical protocol or swallowing a pill. You will need to take substantial steps on your own toward preventing future physical breakdown as well as proper steps to influence the process of healing when you are stricken with disease. This practical awareness of your responsibility to restore and maintain health is also God's gift, one that you need to be willing to accept. It is reasonable to think of your own responsibility to restore and maintain health and wholeness as *self-assisted* healing.

There is much that you can do for yourself—and must do. If you think about it, you live in a "mechanism" of flesh and blood, which you expect to perform flawlessly, sometimes in spite of how you treat it. You expect it to help you achieve the things in life that you hope will bring you success. There is more, of course.

Because you are designed by the Creator for relationship with Him, you must recognize the truth of His Word, which describes the body as "a temple for God" (1 Cor. 6:19–20). That means we are responsible to live in such a way that His presence is comfortable and at home in us. Conscientious care, respect, admiration, and appreciation for the gift of life He has given you leave you with a responsibility. It is up to you—and you alone—to care for your body in positive ways while avoiding harmful elements and taking proper steps to counteract, or reverse, the onset of illness.

The body, with its sixty trillion cells and cellular memory equal to the content of two hundred New York phone books, needs committed attention. There is only one way to have an awareness of the immense responsibility of caring for your body and to accept that responsibility wholeheartedly. It involves appreciating the Creator's intelligent design for your body and thanking Him for life itself. Living in that realization, you will be inspired to assist in the processes of maintaining health and assist in your own restoration to wholeness when sickness strikes. With genuine gratitude and wonder for who you are and what you have received at the Creator's hand, you really have no choice except to take that responsibility.

Your body is not something alien to you. It is the only "house" in which you can live!

PHYSICAL ALIGNMENT

> Do not be deceived, God is not mocked; for whatever a man sows, that he will also reap. For he who sows to his flesh will of the flesh reap corruption, but he who sows to the Spirit will of the Spirit reap everlasting life. And let us not grow weary while doing good, for in due season we shall reap if we do not lose heart.
>
> —GALATIANS 6:7–9

You can help maintain physical balance in your body by promoting the good and minimizing the bad. Health care costs are rising disproportionately to other costs. The last hundred years have seen the primary causes of death shift from consequences of trauma and infection to degenerative diseases such as cancer and arteriosclerosis, diseases that are mediated by lifestyle and therefore preventable.[1] Obesity has now overtaken cancer as the number one preventable cause of death in our country. Attitudes are beginning to change, and health care practitioners are becoming more aware that "the nutritionists of today are the doctors of tomorrow."[2]

Western medicine as a discipline is the practice of science alone to effect cure. As I mentioned, *healing*, as opposed to cure, involves restoring balance: body, soul, and spirit. *Self-assisted* healing indicates the role that patients must assume in order to restore and maintain wholeness in their entire beings. Many patients want the doctor to take control, not only of their healing process but in essence of their destinies, while they remain passive to their self-destructive activities and attitudes of life. Healing requires that you, as a patient, not only heed the advice of physicians but recognize your own responsibility and role in your effecting your healing. This is a magnificent revelation that can help you change your life for the better and ensure that the cure the doctor provides will bring the healing and wholeness you need.

PREVENTION OF DISEASE

> An ounce of prevention is worth a pound of cure.[3]

Ben Franklin's familiar maxim has always been true but never been more to the point than in our present era. It expresses the most powerful aspects of your efforts to assist in your own healing: having proper habits, creating balance and awareness, and making wise choices. The greatest contribution that you can make to your own healing is a commitment to, and work toward, the *prevention* of illness.

What does this mean? It means eating healthy foods and drinking healthy drinks, avoiding dangerous or nutritionally empty foods and substances, making regular exercise a habit, maintaining flourishing relationships, and cultivating a positive attitude. And, more importantly, mostly it means remaining in awe of God's wonderful creation—your body—and respecting it as His handiwork, protecting it as its steward, and remaining faithfully thankful for it. That can only occur as you seek to know your Creator as your Savior, Lord, and intimate friend. In that relationship you will seek to fulfill the purpose for which you were designed. His love will fill you with positive attitudes, lead you into flourishing relationships, and cause you to desire a healthy lifestyle.

HEALTH AND WHOLENESS

The study of health and wholeness touches more profound dimensions of life than most of us think. Although the words *health* and *wholeness* are familiar to everyone, most of us begin the journey to health and restoration very far from ever having known what it means to be physically, mentally, emotionally, and spiritually whole.[4] Wholeness cannot be defined entirely by one visit to the doctor, the introduction to a fad diet, embracing one exercise philosophy, or any other single discipline—total health is multifactorial. But there is a simple answer for many, if not most, health problems; many times you can change the state of your health by simply changing what you put into your system.

Proper nutrition

"It is clear that our Western diet has some serious problems associated with it. Every year, national organizations and government agencies issue dietary guidelines that seem to grow closer and closer to the dietary guidelines God gave to Moses in the Old Testament thousands of years ago. It is no accident that God's wisdom for eating for our health is being 'confirmed' by the latest scientific findings."[5]

Choice of diet is a vital aspect of how you protect yourself. You need to know what your body needs for health and be willing to select those foods that promote health. And you need the self-discipline to deny yourself the foods that break health down. While there are no magical formulas, and what works for some people doesn't work for others, it seems that nutritional supplements, such as vitamins, do provide a healthy addition to enhance a healthful diet.

According to some leaders in the medical field, the best diet is probably a vegetarian diet. That is a diet high in complex carbohydrates and significantly lacking substantial amounts of animal fat. Not only are animal fats to be limited to maintain health but also processed foods, which are traditionally high in salt, sugar, and the empty calories of white flours. Beyond that most of us are well aware these days that substances such as drugs, cigarettes, alcohol, and caffeine must be avoided to promote health in our tissues. You should always drink plenty of water as well.

In the Bible blood is symbolic of the salvation Jesus accomplished on the cross. Blood is also the very real issue of life in our bodies. We need to keep our blood healthy. This is accomplished through balance. Blood must be prone neither to deficiency in quantity (anemia) nor to overabundance (polycythemia). Tempting sweets must be balanced with the proper vitamins and useful nutrients. Moderation and balance are the keys.

Exercise

Start your self-assisted healing with exercise. Our bodies and minds need exercise. How often have you heard this? It is now known that you can best protect your body from disease with exercise. Exercise is a neuro-protector. It protects all the important connections between systems in your body. I used to run to work, twelve miles a day. It was undoubtedly good exercise for me but perhaps not the wisest exercise. It would have been better for me to do interval exercises, using every component of my body, as well as include days designated for rest. A program that includes stretching, interval training, the utilization of all muscles, and plenty of rest is the kind that provides the all-important balance.

A typical daily workout needs to consist of three sections: the warm-up, the main set, and the cooldown. The warm-up and cooldown are important, though often overlooked, aspects. While most of the "work" is accomplished in the main set, the warm-up and cooldown help prevent injury and soreness and allow maximum performance. Strength training—with weights—is as important as any other aspect of training. In weight training remember that full range of motion is vital, as are the order of exercises, proper technique, and breathing.

Developing and maintaining flexibility are extremely important elements in total health. Flexibility decreases after age fifteen, but it can be regained at any age with some effort. Improving flexibility demands focused attention and patience. This is accomplished through stretching the muscles and paying attention to your breathing while doing it.

Complementary methods

These methods apply primarily to our use when we have already fallen ill. The word *healing* can be found in reference to the typical practice of medicine and health care, but it is more commonly applied to what has been called "alternative medicine." In their present "incarnation"—that is, medical methods of healing recognized as an adjunct to traditional, physician-based care—these methods of healing are perhaps more accurately labeled "complementary medicine." The dominant strand in complementary techniques for health and healing involves a personal engagement in the enterprise.

This move from conventional medicine may indicate some disillusionment with conventional approaches, an expression of greater independence, and a growing concern for natural methods that appeal to the whole organism. Still, complementary medicine has recently evolved in a way that is indicative of its ability to *enhance* rather than *replace* the science of modern, conventional medicine.

Some of these techniques may work or help to some degree; others are not scientifically sound; others are simply scams for monetary gain. Alternative methods may seem simpler to understand or at least be more accessible and comprehensible to the patients' intuitive senses—and to their commitment to some sort of action as a means to the end. The more productive and reputable alternative techniques should be included in patients' health protocol as part of their self-assisted healing.

GOD'S WISDOM FOR HEALTH CONFIRMED BY SCIENCE

We live in a culture that is buried under books, gimmicks, and gadgets aimed at diet, fitness, and well-being. However, in this chapter you have become aware that you have a personal role to play in maintaining the strength and vitality of your own body. The human body is equipped with a marvelous defense system that is able to repel or overcome almost every major disease or sickness under normal circumstances. Medical research studies are confirming in increasing numbers and frequency that a healthy diet and regular exercise play a major role in the body's long-term resistance to debilitating disease and sickness. There is more than enough information available to help you assist in your own healing process. Make the choice today to become a willing, active participant in your own healing.

What we eat and what we do with our bodies at every moment alter our bodies at the molecular level. Every choice you make is a block in a foundation for a good life in days, years, decades ahead. Thus the essential attribute of self-assisted healing is personal responsibility. I am responsible for the way I find myself today, I am responsible for the choices I am making today, and therefore, I am responsible for how I will find myself "tomorrow." Goals must be set, but reasonable, achievable ones. Understand that change can be slow; patience will stand you in a better position to adapt. Habits must be developed so that there is no personal conflict.

God's wisdom is a pathway to health and wholeness for you that is paved with wise choices and decisions.

CONCLUSION

"In every area of life, including…food and lifestyle choices and human relationships, my first accountability is to the Word of God. Everything and everybody else need to line up behind that rock-solid source of truth" that assures my health and wholeness.[6]

Illness is a life experience that we share in our lives with each other. Moving like ripples on the surface of a pond, the effects of sickness in one life nudge other lives all around in personal or vicarious suffering. You may be ill yourself or you may be watching your sister or child or friend hurting; in that way each of you participates in the suffering together.

The fact that you picked up this book with interest means that you are already aware that the experience of illness, yours or someone's you love, is not an easy one to face. You may have found it to be unusually deeply troubling and disturbing. It is painful—in many different ways and on several levels. Yet this suffering also has much to teach us.

In reality we are all related to one another on some level as people who are traveling through this life together. This ambient human environment in which we are embedded becomes an integral aspect of our healing. Although it may seem to be a reasonable or obvious point pertaining to health and healing, too often it is neglected in discussions on promoting wholeness for our human race.

As I have mentioned, the question of healing turns on more than just the cessation of pain. Our more profound experiences of illness can point us closer to the truth of who we are as our Creator's unique design. It is in the most difficult episodes of your life that you can learn to see and appreciate the Creator's design, plan, and concern for your existence and prosperity. We are the beneficiaries of a gift of life that is of inestimable value. We are the recipients of a divine design for life, with potential for health and wholeness, as well as eternal destiny bound within the fragile membranes of our cells.

Illness is, unfortunately, an inevitable vulnerability for the human body. During times of illness an enduring appreciation of God's precious gift of life and His desire for eternal relationship with each of us will demand that we seek help to restore health. Through genuine gratefulness for your gift of life from your Creator, along with your awareness of your need for restored health, you can begin your search to make that a reality. The collective knowledge you need to assist in finding your pathway to wholeness will include doctors, nurses, and researchers, as well as neighbors, family, and your responsibility for self-assisted healing. In His great love for us God has provided all we need to live a life in intimate relationship with Him and learn to walk in health and wholeness in His love and wisdom.

DISCUSSION QUESTIONS

List the preventative measures you incorporate into your lifestyle to maintain health and wholeness in your mind, body, and spirit.

Regardless of what you've done in the past, what new steps can you take to incorporate more healthy choices into your lifestyle?

Write a scripture that will help you focus on the importance of making healthy choices.

CHAPTER 6

GOD'S Rx FOR **YOUR ALIGNMENT**

IN THE NEXT chapters, we will discuss issues concerning ways for your body, mind, and spirit to come into alignment with God's Rx for health and wholeness. We will also consider hindrances that may keep you from finding your godly pathway to wholeness in any of those areas. Balance and healthy alignment with the original purpose of the Creator of life for your entire being requires a journey into relationship with Him, one that He purposed for you from the beginning. That heart journey is the most rewarding, satisfying path of life you will ever discover. And it is God's desire to draw you into that journey with Him by His great love for you.

Together we have thought about the wisdom of God in creation, who embedded in the DNA of every person the alignment pattern for wholeness in His intelligent design. We looked at the body's natural ability to preserve balance and to reestablish that balance on occasions when it is lost. All the appropriate reactions to injury that are required for physical healing are founded on these principles for healing imbedded within your body.

You are a recipient of this divine gift of innate healing for your body from the Lord. It is your appreciation and respect for your design, as well as for the designer, that requires that you seek the pathway to health and wholeness for your life. By making a personal commitment to constantly take care of your body, you may be able to prevent imbalances and illness in the first place. This commitment also involves your decisions to make significant alterations in personal behavior that may have caused an upset in balance that leads to illness or disease.

In the earlier chapters we also discussed the occasions of imbalance and ill health that will require the assistance of doctors. Biological life, for a human, is incredibly complex. For that reason freedom from illness and pain cannot always be realized without some kind of professional medical intervention beyond your own natural resources and efforts. When you find yourself in that situation, you need to prayerfully trust the health professionals to discern the Creator's intended process of healing for you that will restore equilibrium and completeness to your body.

Professional medical people are equipped to employ methods of healing borne of the wisdom discovered by science in the Creator's physical design for mankind. This skill and understanding with which physicians, researchers, health scientists, and clinicians are endowed are God's second gift of healing to us, after the innate healing embedded in the body at creation.

For many of us that innate source of healing through the wonders of our bodies, along with our attentive stewardship to our bodies for prevention of sickness, is our major source of health maintenance. Then, if sickness strikes, the caring assistance of medical experts is our next recourse for restoration of health. Yet as helpful as those resources for restoring health are, do they exhaust the definition of and possibilities for our restoration to wholeness? Is all healing a physical event that occurs as a result of these healing resources?

Put another way, are there situations of loss of health that cannot be resolved by the healing resources we have discussed?

Perhaps you have suffered your own wrenching experience of illness in which your beautiful inner self has been twisted by pain that no physician can resolve. Or consider the tragedy of a parent losing a child to leukemia. Or watching a dear friend descend into pits of despair and decay. And in the issue of life and death how do we personally approach our own mortality, our understanding of eternity? What direction can we choose as a pathway to restore alignment for health of body, mind, and spirit in these and other difficult situations?

People are so much more than physical clumps of tissues or a reflection of the results of their labor and achievements. We are not simply physical entities as cod fish and fir trees are. We are physical, mental, emotional, and spiritual beings. All aspects of the exceptionally designed human body are integrated into a unified whole, which is infinitely greater than the sum of its parts. Indeed, observing the completeness and beauty of the entire person mirrors this profound reality. So how do illness and healing reveal alignment, or the lack of it, consciously within your *inner* being? Your mind? Your emotions? Your spirit?

The healthy unification of all elements that make up our humanity requires establishing balance and communication among body, mind, emotions, and spirit. Wholeness and balance at the mental and spiritual levels have been proved to affect the capacity of your physical body to heal. As a thinking, feeling, created being made in the image of your Creator, you have profound need for mental and spiritual alignment when balance has been overturned in those areas.

What is required for this healing and restoration of mind and spirit to become a reality? What are the ways you can seek to create balance within yourself in order to be healed? To experience wholeness? What is God's prescription for your inner realignment that will establish health again?

God's Word tells us that we need to be transformed in our thinking as we become aligned with Christ, receiving Him as our Savior in order to be the recipients of all that He is. It takes full surrender of our lives to God to engage this integration of God into all that we are: body, soul, and spirit. We will need to pray as Christ did in Gethsemane: "Not my will, but Yours, be done" (Luke 22:42). This total consecration of your life to God makes you a holy, pleasing, and available recipient of all He is, including His "realignment" of your body, mind, and spirit to His design.

As you receive God's love and forgiveness and enter into a spiritual journey with Christ, you will discover a life of continual healing—health and wholeness—spiritually as well as physically. God made us to live in harmony with Him in order for every aspect of our beings to dwell in wholeness. It is this fellowship with God, for which you were created, that will release you into His divine health. Not only physically but in your inner being you will bask in His love, learning to rest in His redemption: His peace, joy, and righteousness.

When we were speaking of physical health and healing, we were referring to maintaining or reacquiring balance by adhering to guidelines that the body's design dictates. To achieve this physical wholeness, you align yourself with God's purpose by accepting the stewardship of your temple in which He will dwell. Then, regarding wholeness of hearts and minds, we are referencing the prosperity that comes to your inner being as you embrace the spiritual principles and precepts through which alignment with God was established in creation. As your body, mind, and spirit come into harmony with God's design and His plan, realignment will be complete and wholeness, restored.

For example, to be realigned mentally with God's design, you must seek to have "the mind of Christ" (1 Cor. 2:16), remain positive and hopeful, and constantly rejoice with great feelings of thankfulness. For realignment to be achieved spiritually, you must allow God's Holy Spirit to reign in every area of your life. And by focusing on eternal life with God rather than temporal existence in this world as your priority, you will be realigned with God and His purposes for your life (2 Cor.

4:16–18). In short, inner healing is the healing of mind and spirit through realignment to God's will for your life. When this happens, your body is also strengthened through that harmony and heart relationship you are developing with Christ.

MIND AND BODY—BODY AND MIND

Intuitively you are aware that you are not made up of "divided" portions of body, mind, and spirit; each of these areas of your life is profoundly connected, each a part of a singularity and therefore each deeply influencing the others. Those influences are more profound than you may know, however. Science is just now teasing out the details of the depth of the relationships among body, mind, and spirit. For example, recent research indicates that emotional pain excites the same parts of the brain as physical pain does and as strongly.

As we have discussed, some illnesses heal under the energies of the body's natural systems. Some require medical intervention, while the healing of others can be accomplished through diet, exercise, and lifestyle changes. And yet other illnesses can be attributed to one's mental and spiritual states. Errant emotions, fears, and anxieties can kill. Only the realignment of your inner self can assist in restoring your overall well-being.

Numerous studies have now pointed out the weighty influence of the mind-body connection. We are being increasingly informed about the role of depression, loneliness, unhappiness, fear, and anger in the development and prolongation of diseases such as cancer, heart disease, diabetes, and asthma.[1] *Mind* refers to the complete array of "mental functions related to thinking, mood, and purposive behavior. The mind is generally seen as deriving from activities in the brain but displaying emergent properties, such as consciousness."[2]

Typically we think of the mind as centered in the brain. Scientific research indicates that our thoughts and feelings influence the body through two primary "channels": the nervous system and the circulatory system.[3] The brain, as the center of the nervous system, sends and receives electrical impulses from every part of the body. You can move a toe under the brain's instructions, and that toe also "tells" your brain, you, when it has struck something painfully. Significantly, with nerve endings in the bone marrow (the birthplace of white cells), the brain influences the mighty immune system. In addition, your brain is a gland that secretes hormones that affect the entire endocrine system.

Just how deep the mind-body connection is remains somewhat of a mystery; however, every physician knows about the reality of the "placebo effect." A placebo is an inert, virtually useless substance (a sugar pill, if you will) sometimes administered to a patient (normally in trials for new medications) under the pretense that it is a powerful drug that will directly improve their condition. Results from the administration of placebos have indeed demonstrated improvement or "healing" in statistically significant numbers of patients. Likewise, upon learning that their "medicine" was not what they believed it to be, some patients have experienced a reversion to their original sickness. There is no explanation for this outside of the influence of thought and feelings on the whole person. You have heard the adage "You are what you eat." You are also *what you think*.

The implications are so marked that some refer to it as the "biology of belief."[4] This intertwining of influence among body, mind, and spirit has dramatic effects on our overall health. It is in the body, with its strengths and weaknesses; the brain/mind, with its thoughts, feelings, and consciousness; and the spirit, with committed trust in God and communion with Him, that health and wholeness can be ultimately restored to our entire person. It all began with God's intention out of His heart of love to create you in His image to become a son or daughter in Him—forever.

MENTAL HEALTH AND WHOLENESS

It has been observed that hopelessness breeds recklessness—or we might use the term *imbalance*. And to enjoy mental health, we must have balance through faith and reason. This necessary balance for mental health derives from an understanding and appreciation of the Creator's wisdom. It is as we cultivate an intimate relationship with our God through faith in Christ that we gain this appreciation of God's wisdom regarding our lives.

Without that wisdom people may seek escape from life's difficult challenges and emotional pain through the use of damaging substances and the practice of harmful behaviors. That unhealthy retreat into self-destructive compulsions and addictions is frequently seen as a substitute for the rest and relief that God offers to every person who receives Him in redemption. That kind of false retreat from life's suffering is a grave mistake. Those errant behaviors only complicate things, damage health, and further alienate our hearts from ourselves, our Creator, and our divine purpose.

When you are faced with illness, you are presented with something that might very well be life changing in a variety of ways. But in a positive light through that illness you are afforded the opportunity to contemplate your life and to discover personal transformation and growth. You will ask, "How can I make sense of what is happening? How can I remain hopeful? How can I live?" when you are weak and the negative emotion of fear becomes your primary sense. How do you face death? How do you face life? Who you are and how you face trouble are so important. These and other questions, when directed to your loving heavenly Father, can bring you to an understanding of His love and purpose for you that can bring transformation to your life.

HOPE AND WHOLENESS

Biology plays a large part in the development of your personality, as do the social environments you are exposed to from birth. In addition, however, we also have personal choices to make. For example, we can choose how we face our challenges in life, either in a despairing attitude or in choosing to live in hope. You and I must learn to appreciate the designer of life and our design, and decide how we will relate to Him. When we accept His invitation to become His sons and daughters through the power of the Holy Spirit and faith in Christ, He begins to give us true understanding of the center of control in our lives. In that relationship of divine love we have power to choose hope over hostility and all negative emotions. Prayer and faith in God have been demonstrated to be catalysts to lower levels of hostility and raise levels of hope.

Dr. James Avery works with hospice patients, those who are dying and will not ever get better. He believes that not only is hope a real possibility in one's last days, but it is also a necessity.[5] It's true, the hopes of those facing imminent death largely differ from those people who are still living healthy lives. Those facing imminent death hope for a peaceful death, share hopes for loved ones left, and even hope for a healing that beats the odds—but the important thing is that hope flowers in every heart, bringing peace and rest.

It is vital that we comprehend the immensity of this power of hope. As Dutch Sheets writes, "Hope deferred is the common cold of the soul, except that this virus can kill."[6] Our Creator endowed us with the inner capacity for hope; it is part of His design for healing. We must nurture it in ourselves and encourage it in one another. The power of hope in the process of healing is as important as any medication, treatment, or nutrient.

Perhaps you are familiar with the biblical story of Joseph, the son of the patriarch Jacob who was betrayed by his brothers, sold into slavery, and later thrown into prison. During a terrible famine, his brothers encountered him as a ruler in Egypt, in charge of all the food they desperately needed. Joseph wept over his brothers and reassured them that though they had meant their actions for evil, "God meant it for good" to provide for them during the famine (Gen. 50:20). Joseph's perspective allowed him to live in hope, knowing that God can only do what is good for those who love and trust Him. He faced years of hardship without losing hope in his relationship with God. As humans, we cannot live without hope, without the sense that something good can result from our deepest tragedy. There are many ways that even illness may end produce something good in our lives as we submit to God even in our difficult time. Your ability to hope, to search for God's plan within the hardship, is a central key to healing and restoration to wholeness.

CAN HOPE BE A CURE?

Faith gives substance to hope (Heb. 11:1). Hope is important, but hope lacks substance until it is rooted in FAITH: fully assured I trust Him! Hope is faith talking aloud, drowning out voices of defeat. An example is found in Mark 5:25–28, where the woman with the issue of blood said, "If only I may touch His clothes, I shall be made well." Hope gave her the tenacity to press forward in faith. The Amplified Bible, Classic Edition says, "For she kept saying, If I only touch His garments, I shall be restored to health."

Hope is birthed in an attitude of gratitude that causes you to expect joyously even if you have to wait for the answer. When you are assured of the character of God, you can develop a habit of thankfulness toward God and others. That grateful heart puts you into a frame of mind to expect to receive blessing and enjoy life in the future. Conversely, cynicism and criticism squelch hope and faith within a heart. They may be rooted in some resentment and bitterness that have not been repented of. These negative attitudes will barricade your way to health and keep you from going forward into wholeness.

Your words are "seeds" that will bring a harvest. Words of hope will bring a wonderful harvest to your own life. And you can energize others with words of hope and encouragement even in your own trying times. "Death and life are in the power of the tongue" (Prov. 18:21). Regardless of what your circumstances are, as you yield your life to God, you are learning to rest in the character of God—He never fails.

The Bible records that Abraham hoped against hope when he was old and no longer physically able to bring forth the heir God had promised him and his wife, Sarah (Rom. 4:18). It isn't human nature to hope against hope. In fact such a response seems contrary to human sanity, but an irrepressible trust in God is always rewarded. (See Romans 4:13–25.) The peace of God surpasses our understanding and human reasoning (Phil. 4:6–7). Joyous faith founded in hope cannot be explained, but it is steadfastly based on "the substance of things hoped for, the evidence of things not [yet] seen" (Heb. 11:1; see also 1 Pet. 1:7–8). Hope breaks us out of the net of reasoning and moves us forward in faith and confidence in God and His Word. Hope renews our minds.

Hebrews 6:18–19 tells us that when disappointment and confusion come, our response should be to run to the Lord, not sink into despair. God's faithfulness in times past enables us to hope again and to pass this hope along to others. Hope is "an anchor of the soul, both sure and steadfast" (v. 19).

As we receive God's Word through faith, hope rises within us. When we live it out before others as "living epistles," those who see our witness receive His living, life-giving hope just as they receive it by reading His written epistles. Their faith in Him will be enhanced when we are anchored in Him! In the times in which we live, Christians, anchored in the rock, Christ Jesus, will be able to extend a hand of hope to those terrorized by the current events that are sure to happen before Jesus returns.

> Why art thou cast down, O my soul? and why art thou disquieted in me? hope thou in God: for I shall yet praise him for the help of his countenance.
>
> —Psalm 42:5, KJV

It is the powerful, living Word of God applied by the power of the Holy Spirit in the name of Jesus to any situation that quickens the life-changing promises of God. As long as you are content with a thimbleful of God, you will only view life from the standpoint of reports of illness, bad relationship scenarios, and hopeless circumstances, and your soul will be troubled as a result. But when you hope in God and His Word, it will transform you into a man or woman of faith. The Word of God comes alive in you when you call upon the Holy Spirit of God to awaken your spirit and soul to who God is. Jeremiah 32:17 reminds you: "There is nothing too hard for thee" (KJV). In that heart that is yielded to the truth of God's Word, hope *can* become a cure as you say with the psalmist:

> Why are you cast down, O my soul? And why are you disquieted within me? Hope in God, for I shall yet praise Him for the help of His countenance.
>
> —Psalm 42:5

DISCUSSION QUESTIONS

Describe a person or situation in your life that brought you hope. Did that hope last, or was it temporary?

What does *hope* mean to you?

Write a scripture that reminds you of the hope you have in Christ.

CHAPTER 7

THE ROLE OF FAITH IN GOD'S Rx

CLINICAL EVIDENCE SHOWS and formal studies have been conducted that confirm the positive influence of a religious faith on healing. This includes the positive effects of fellowship and worship attendance at church, of private religious activities such as daily devotional prayer, and of intercessory prayer (individuals praying for the healing of other people). So positive are these effects that health practitioners are finding faith difficult to ignore.[1] These research studies have been published in a variety of medical journals.[2]

Statistics reported by WebMD give the following indications for people who do not attend church or profess a faith in God:

- Their average hospital stays are longer than the hospital stays for believers.
- They are several times more likely to die following surgery.
- They have a 40 percent higher death rate from heart disease and cancer.
- They experience twice the number of strokes.[3]

In this chapter we will take a closer look at some of these expressions of religious faith meant to encourage you to seek God's blessing and healing in all you do.

PRAYER

> Is anyone among you sick? Let him call for the elders of the church, and let them pray over him, anointing him with oil in the name of the Lord. And the prayer of faith will save the sick, and the Lord will raise him up.
>
> —James 5:14–15

The most widely cited study to date on the therapeutic effects of prayer was conducted by Dr. Randolph Byrd at the San Francisco Medical Center in 1988. Dr. Byrd studied a coronary care unit (CCU) population to explore two questions:

1. Does intercessory prayer to the Judeo-Christian God have any effect on the patient's medical condition and recovery while in the hospital?
2. How are these effects characterized, if present?[4]

In this study 393 patients were assigned randomly to one of two groups. Group 1 had prayers made to God on behalf of the patients by intercessors. Group 2, the control group, received no prayers from anyone associated with the study. Intercessory prayer for each member in the first group was exercised by three to seven intercessors, who were provided with the patient's name and diagnosis, and information on the patient's general condition. Intercessors selected were born-again Christians with active Christian lives in their churches. All 393 patients received the same high-quality cardiac care at the hospital. The identities of the individuals in each group were kept secret from the attending doctors, nurses, and patients themselves.

Dr. Byrd recorded the dramatic results of his statistical study about the efficacy of remote intercessory prayer.

> Analysis of events after entry into the study showed the prayer group had less congestive heart failure, required less diuretic and antibiotic therapy, had fewer episodes of pneumonia, had fewer cardiac arrests, and were less frequently intubated and ventilated.[5]

Dr. Byrd concluded that with intercessory prayer to God—from a distance and without the beneficiary's knowledge—"there seemed to be an effect, and that effect was presumed to be beneficial."[6]

In another study of patients suffering from rheumatoid arthritis (RA), the authors reported that individuals receiving in-person intercessory prayer—prayer with direct contact between the intercessor and the patient—showed significant improvement in their one-year follow-up.[7] The researchers concede that further explorations are required with more detailed examination of possible placebo effects, as well as the "varying types and degrees of spiritual and religious beliefs and practices." However, their study already suggests that "in-person intercessory prayer may be a useful adjunct to standard medical care for certain patients with rheumatoid arthritis."[8]

This conclusion of this study is an important point. William Standish Reed, founder of the Christian Medical Foundation, surgeon, scholar, and strong believer, made it clear.

> I believe implicitly in the Healing Ministry of the Church of Jesus Christ. However, I believe that the ministry should be used in conjunction with the best medical and surgical methods—not as a substitute for scientific methods. It is my belief that the answer to the prayer of the cancer sufferers often is the scalpel of the well-trained surgeon.[9]

Other researchers have noted statistically significant beneficial effects of immersion in a personal and private practice of Christian faith. In one study the researchers sought to reveal an association between private religious activities (meditation, prayer, or Bible study) and longer survival in certain groups.[10] Establishing controls for demographics and health status, the researchers reported that among community-dwelling adults aged 64–101, "persons with no disability and little or no private religious activity ... were 63 percent more likely to die" over the six-year period of the study. "Even after controlling for social support and health behaviors, investigators found that lack of private religious activity continued to predict a 47 percent greater risk of dying."[11]

Another hospital study of cardiac patients, this one in 1999 at St. Luke's Hospital of Kansas City, found that a group of patients who received daily prayer from Christian volunteers had "shorter recovery times with fewer complications" than the group that received no prayer. William Harris, PhD, who conducted the study, concluded that "prayer may be an effective adjunct to standard medical care."[12]

Dr. Larry Dossey makes that point even more stridently. He states that "if the subject of [Byrd's] study had been a new medication instead of prayer, this would have been considered a medical breakthrough. Up until then most medical people had considered prayer a nice thing. It didn't hurt much, but they certainly didn't consider it a matter of life and death."[13]

Dossey wisely points out that "when we talk of prayer we are talking about distant manifestations of consciousness. To talk this way is to break some kind of taboo. We can accept the power of the mind in affecting bodily processes, but to talk interpersonally—that my consciousness can have an effect on other persons and events—is a major paradigm shift."[14]

Harold G. Koenig notes that the work of others has indicated the possible mechanisms of religion's action or influence on health—on hypertension, in this case. The beneficial effect of religion on blood pressure is most likely a combination of factors that include:

- The promotion of healthy lifestyle practices
- Coping effects of religious practice
- Social support effects of integration into a religious community
- Beneficial psychodynamics of particular belief systems and faith[15]

When you are baffled and desperate for an answer to life, the Holy Spirit can lead you to prayer that is "according to the will of God" (Rom. 8:27). Jesus Himself taught us to pray, "Thy kingdom come, Thy will be done in earth, as it is in heaven" (Matt. 6:10, KJV). When we pray in agreement with the will of God, we know that all heaven is on our side. What a comfort to know that when we ask anything according to God's will, He hears us and grants the things that we ask (1 John 5:14–15).

The apostle Paul admonished us to "pray without ceasing" (1 Thess. 5:17). How is this possible? When you wake up at night, think of His love for you and not of the world and its anxieties. Be constantly thinking about your Redeemer and about your relationship with Him as you go through your days. Staying in close contact with God will help you when the rough spots in your life occur. He is just a call away.

> Call to Me, and I will answer you, and show you great and mighty things, which you do not know.
>
> —Jeremiah 33:3

What I refer to as "breath prayers" have become a true blessing and a refreshing way to go through the busy workday at our clinic. These prayers are short and simple requests, spoken in one breath. They can be one phrase of praise, gratitude, or worship. Try your own breath prayers—they will help you cope with whatever situations arise in your day. They certainly will remind you of God's continual grace in your daily life. After all, it is His very breath that you are breathing that gives and sustains your life.

Here are some breath prayers you can use daily:

- "Give me gentleness, Father."
- "Bring healing to this patient, Father; guide me in my part."
- "Bless my children, their spouses, and my grandchildren today, Father."
- "Help me better understand and live Your truth today."
- "May I live for the anointing, Father; it's the presence of the Holy One."

Our friend Ralph McIntosh battled an aggravating bout of symptoms, including chest pains, for a few years that the doctors couldn't define well enough to determine the right treatment. At one point he was hospitalized and tests were run, but still there was no conclusive evidence. A resulting weakness drained his strength so much that he had trouble climbing stairs without pulling himself up one step at a time by clinging to the handrails. He knew something was terribly wrong with him, but no test pinpointed the problem.

One day while his wife, Susan, was at work, in desperation he determined to seek the Lord's healing for himself. He pulled two chairs together in their living room and sat down to have a time of focused communion with the Lord. He spoke aloud, "Jesus, am I dying? If so, I want to know so I can get things in order for my wife and family." For some time he sat there waiting for an answer. Then he sensed that he was in the presence of the Lord Jesus, communing with Him person to person. He experienced an amazing spiritual moment with the Lord, and from that day forward Ralph began to get well. The weakness left, and his health returned. With the healing came a renewed purpose and call upon his life. That day he received an inner healing and a spiritual commissioning. Within a few years he gave up his contracting business, and he and his wife went into full-time Christian ministry.

Isaiah had the same reaction in Isaiah 6. Our reaction to His glorious presence is worship followed by a deeper awareness of our need of redemption and a commissioning to tell others of Him. We conclude, "Here am I! Send me" (Isa. 6:8).

FELLOWSHIP

John Donne believed that no man is an island. Many of us live our lives ignoring that simple, difficult truth until we become ill. It is well documented that vibrant social bonds are an integral element in health, healing, and longevity.[16] At St. Luke's we are keenly aware of the beneficial effects that accompany reaching out to the individual patient in a helpful, human, loving manner.

God had good reasons for commanding us to fellowship with one another. There is something about having to "rub elbows" with other people that keeps us from isolating ourselves, especially when we are struggling with emotional issues. Even children today seem far more self-centered than they were years ago when two, three, or more siblings had to share a bedroom. Their continual contact taught them to give in to one another, to enjoy and appreciate them, even to care for the needs of their siblings.

Whether it's a church family, a social club, a gym, a service club, a volunteer position at a hospital, a book club, or a twelve-step support group, relationships provide the exercise of staying in touch with others. Some of the loneliest people wait for their phones or doorbells to ring and complain because no one cares. That is not a healthy perspective of how to interact with others. Not only is it your *responsibility* to reach out to others; it actually is a privilege to be involved with others' lives. Even if you aren't a "group" kind of person, you were created to communicate—and it is that interaction with others that helps keep you healthy.

Healthy relationships are important. Loneliness kills; we should avoid it like the plague. Psychologists at McGill University took a group of heart attack survivors who were being discharged from the hospital and divided them up into two groups. Both groups received the same excellent heart care from the cardiologists and their own family physicians. However, one group also received monthly phone calls from some of the research team members. If the researcher making the phone contact sensed any psychosocial problem, a specially trained nurse was scheduled to visit the patient in the home. Just that little personal contact that was made resulted in a 50 percent reduction in the patients' death rate after one year in the group that was cared for by occasional phone calls and visits.[17]

Stanford researchers randomly assigned women with metastatic breast cancer to receive usual medical care plus a weekly support group designed to help them manage the stress of their illness. The support group patients lived twice as long as those who were not in the program. At UCLA patients with malignant melanoma who participated in only six ninety-minute sessions with a support group that also provided relationship training had a 50 percent reduction in patient death and recurrence of symptoms compared with patients who received the usual care. Over the six years of this study more than three times as many patients in the nonintervention group died compared with the group that received support.[18]

All of us need interaction with others. It causes us to forget about ourselves when we focus on the needs of others. God made us to need one another. We need listening ears, caring hearts, and it must be a two-way street in order for a family, a community, or a church to be made up of healthy, emotionally fulfilled people.

As a Christian you are admonished to encourage others, pray for others, sing together, and testify of what God is doing in your life in order to edify—build up others in Christian love. Your life is enriched when you reach out to others and let them reach out to you. We do live in a fallen world where sin and pain abound. Many times, through no fault of our own, we are victims of "heart wounding." When that happens, our tendency is to pull in to ourselves and avoid close relationships. We think, "If people know this or that about me, they wouldn't like me and won't want to be my friend." This is self-deception that will compound our pain through loneliness.

Fellowship with others is a freeing experience. God has placed distinct gifts and aspects of His divine nature within you. When you fellowship with others, you can edify them with your life. The body of Christ will be complete someday when all of us are together with Him in glory. It is pride that keeps us from humbling ourselves and admitting that we need one another. God created us to need one another. We are incomplete apart from the other members of the body of Christ.

THE "BLESSED" MINDSET

Alignment—the key to inner healing—really involves total abandonment to God and the Holy Spirit reigning within your heart and mind. The Lord created you in a wonderful way, yet the many aspects of your consciousness must be kept in check continually by your proximity to God and His will. Ungodly, destructive, and negative thoughts proclaim that we are bound rather than freed by the Holy Spirit. Developing God's "blessed" mindset is an important step toward true alignment with His design and desire for you. Aligning with God's will by adopting His "blessed" mindset allows us to experience the consequent inner healing that every one of us seeks—whether we are aware of the need or not.

The mental attitudes that produce mental health are those we embrace as we align ourselves with the Creator—and these are outlined most explicitly in the Beatitudes, found in Matthew 5:3–12. They present what I believe is the best summary of God's "blessed" mindset, which is the mindset of inner health. That mindset produces a life that stands in direct opposition to the life produced under a burden of sin.

The first beatitude says, "Blessed are the poor in spirit, for theirs is the kingdom of heaven" (v. 3). Humility is listed as the first requirement for having God's spirit within us. However, we are often preoccupied with self-centeredness and pride. We are concerned with satisfying what we feel are our needs. How am I going to be hurt? What does that person think about me? How does this make me look? What do I get out of this? The mindset described in the beatitudes is one that is centered on God and others—not on self. It is a spirit of humility and God-wardness.

The theme of humility continues in the second beatitude, which pronounces God's blessing on the brokenhearted: "Blessed are those who mourn, for they shall be comforted" (v. 4). Matthew is describing people who know the glory of repentance and forgiveness, as David did in Psalm 51. The Savior has told us that we are blessed when we mourn because we will be comforted in the breast of the Trinity. Life is temporary and therefore involves suffering, but our growing relationship with the triune God is forever. Irrespective of the earthly circumstances we must face, God's authentic healing touch is eternal and ever present.

"Blessed are the meek, for they shall inherit the earth" (Matt. 5:5). The significance of meekness is in learning truly to submit to and abide by the Lord's teachings. The meek are those who fall into alignment with His instructions. Unless we follow Him and abide in His teachings, we will never really have anything.

Meekness is not weakness; it is "controlled strength." Without the revelation of and obedience to what the Lord would have us accomplish, we would be dangerous. Our nature can sometimes tell us to drive ourselves to success or to exact justice on another through our own power. Meekness, however, means living under authority—God's authority. Only there can true justice or success be found.

Pride will destroy us. In our independence of Him we cannot inherit God's portion for us in this life, or the new heavens and the new earth in eternity. But when we abide in Him, we inherit the earth.

"Blessed are those who hunger and thirst for righteousness, for they shall be filled" (v. 6). It is individuals who embrace this fourth beatitude attitude who are pronounced happy and filled! A basic human flaw affecting every person is that we are full of and bound by personal desire. Selfish desires are like thorns that choke the Word of God in our lives. The empty quest to fulfill earthly desire inevitably remains unquenched, merely increasing the yearning for it. Human desire can never be satisfied or fulfilled. It is only as we truly hunger and thirst after God's ways that we will find true satisfaction. Seek after God, and you will find God Himself in the paths of obedience that He has marked out for you in His Word.

The fifth beatitude tells us, "Blessed are the merciful, for they shall obtain mercy" (v. 7). No one is closer to the very heart of Christ Himself than a merciful, forgiving man or woman who is patient with the pains and shortcomings of others. The path to one's own inner healing is to be found as you show mercy in nurturing and assisting the healing of others. A merciful heart lacks traces of bitterness and envy and is distinguished by an unwillingness to hold grudges or aggravate injury. Rather, a merciful mindset allows you to become an intercessor rather than an accuser and counts it a glory to pass by a transgression. Such a happy soul is God's channel of grace in a world full of hate.

The sixth beatitude is given as, "Blessed are the pure in heart, for they shall see God" (v. 8). This is a profound source of encouragement that will keep you moving toward alignment during those difficult times when you find yourself tempted to take a harmful path. Gazing at God's joyful countenance will focus your determination on keeping your heart pure. If you do not keep your eyes on God, you will be aimed toward those things that will ultimately defile you. The devil always shows you the apple but never the worm hidden inside that will destroy you. Many peaceful homes and marriages have been ruined by an eye that was diverted from God. Searching for—and seeing—the face of God, especially during times of temptation, brings spiritual pleasures that are infinitely more satisfying than trying to satiate an earthly appetite. An aligned mind will lead to the spiritual gifts that ennoble and strengthen the soul.

The "peacemakers" have this happy benediction in the seventh beatitude: "Blessed are the peacemakers, for they shall be called sons of God" (v. 9). God's healing is found in the gospel of reconciliation. What a blessing it is to be what Paul calls "God's coworkers" as we seek to unite hard and bitter hearts (1 Cor. 3:9, TLB). Under God's blessing and power people become soft and tender toward one another. Such sweet fellowship is wonderful evidence that God can change the very bent of a soul. Peacemaking is a necessity to experience God's inner healing and peace and to share them.

The final beatitude is pronounced on those who are persecuted for the sake of righteousness. "Blessed are those who are persecuted for righteousness' sake, for theirs is the kingdom of heaven" (v. 10). One of the heaviest weights for the human spirit to bear is to be falsely accused. It is human nature to immediately defend our honor when challenged unfairly, while conveniently forgetting the many times when we were actually in the wrong yet neither caught nor exposed. Such selective sight and memory cause us to defend ourselves with great energy to almost any limit. However, to humbly bear false accusation is to follow the Savior's example. We may be hated, persecuted, or hurt by others for doing what is right in God's eyes. Jesus tells us to rejoice and be exceedingly glad in these cases because He will reward us greatly in heaven.

There is comfort in God's attitude toward us here. This comfort is the foundation of all the beatitudes. We seek to please God and rest in His redemption, content that we know our God and love Him and aim to please Him. This is the blessed mindset in a life aligned with God. This mental alignment frees you from the destructive patterns of thought that ruin your life and relationships and distance you from the Creator. In this alignment you can experience a mindset free to enjoy the liberty that God designed the soul to experience. The beatitudes outline an escape from the selfish patterns of thinking that naturally imprison the mind and heart.

Here is another important key to freedom and inner healing:

> Come aside by yourselves to a deserted place and rest a while.
>
> —Mark 6:31

Jesus offered this invitation to His disciples to seek some rest and refreshment, a break from the noise and labor of life. Inevitably, though, the spiritually hungry multitudes followed them on their escape. Jesus, moved by compassion, taught the eager crowd of more than five thousand and fed them with two fish and five loaves of bread. Finally, after a long day, He drew apart once more for the much-needed peace and solitude that He had not yet been able to find, going alone to the mountain to pray (Mark 6:46).

If Jesus, God's Son, required such quiet times, how much

more do we? Nurturing the spirit of peaceful solitude is part of your healing. Only by recharging yourself are you ever going to be capable of helping and loving others when faced with their needs and demands. You need silence to hear God's voice.

In Jerusalem there was a very special pool where "lay a great multitude of sick people, blind, lame, paralyzed, waiting for the moving of the water" (John 5:3). The pool of Bethesda (lit. house of mercy) drew those seeking healing. It provided cooling waters to those living in the middle of the city. This pool of Bethesda was a great mercy to the people of Jerusalem for its healing and restorative powers through God's grace.

The anguish and neuroses that we feel so deeply at times arise out of too much time we have spent overly focused upon ourselves. We tend to exaggerate our discomforts rather than enjoying peace and anointing. To dip in the pool is to dispense with all of your preoccupation with pain and simply rest in the Lord's arms. This is where you find physical, mental, and spiritual healing. You need to establish in your life a deserted place or a pool of healing in which to rest regularly in quiet communion with your God in His Word and in prayer.

God's Word is a profound source of rest and restoration, for it is there that faith and grace abide. (See Chapter 10.) There, under God's sovereign hand, can be found every promise of God, sufficient for all your healings. Your place of rest may also include the place of prayer, meditation, and reflection upon God's gorgeous creation. Perhaps a simple walk on the beach or in the mountains is all that is necessary from time to time for you to slow down, relax, and reorient yourself to the Lord.

Wherever it may be, be sure you find a "deserted place" (Mark 6:31) that will afford you the rest of calm and quiet—your pool of Bethesda. We live in a world of temptation, paranoia, confusion, chaos, and turmoil. Resting in a quiet place, with the Lord as the object of your focus, you will triumph.

If you try to manage your difficulties separated from Him, out of alignment with His way, you will fail. The effects of such spiritual alignment with God are equivalent to a healing; losses incurred by neglecting this alignment are eternal.

How do you use your free time? What do most people do in their time outside their forty- to sixty-hour workweeks? Do they sit in front of the TV or hang out with the boys? What do you do? Many activities are meaningful, and many more merely seem meaningful. In the long run what judges the activity is whether you grow stronger or weaker through it. Well-used free time helps you get into condition physically, mentally, and spiritually. Time spent properly can refresh you and send you back into life rejuvenated.

During their free time many people become bored, which leads frequently to a self-centered lifestyle rather than an abundant life. A self-centered lifestyle leads down the short, slippery slope to spiritual blindness. In that state you will begin to worry about everything rather than offering the Creator thanksgiving for the blessings of this life. Make judicious use of your free time. Instead of thinking constantly about yourself, look on the needs of others and ways you can become a help, a friend, and encouragement for another. "Therefore we do not lose heart. Even though our outward man is perishing, yet the inward man is being renewed day by day" (2 Cor. 4:16).

The abundant life can be experienced only after we have learned to rejoice and be thankful. "Rejoice in the Lord always. Again I will say, rejoice!" (Phil. 4:4). Don't waste your time in this life; it is your preparation for eternity. The Word tells you to "be anxious for nothing, but in everything by prayer and supplication, with thanksgiving, let your requests be made known to God" (Phil. 4:6). This is what is most important—praying, meditating, appreciating, and doing. "The things which you learned and received and heard and saw in me, these do, and the God of peace will be with you" (Phil 4:9). Such a mindset is applicable to your activities twenty-four hours a day. Simply listening to what you ought to do, or even understanding what you ought to do, is insufficient. You are required to do what God has purposed for you to do—and to do it with a thankful heart.

The purpose of aligning your mind with God's purposes is to be restored to wholeness and to experience the unction of God—that is, His presence and power—living within you. You cannot experience His presence in this way without quiet, personal times spent in His presence.

DISCUSSION QUESTIONS

Has your faith ever had a positive impact on your physical health? Your mental health?

What symptoms are you experiencing that might be eliminated by strengthening your faith?

What is the first step you will take toward strengthening your faith?

CHAPTER 8

HINDRANCES TO SPIRITUAL ALIGNMENT

In the previous chapter we saw the necessity of the power of faith working in our hearts to help to realign us with God spiritually. As we saw, the beatitudes Jesus taught are a beautiful description of and powerful instruction for a life spiritually aligned with God's heart and character of love. In this chapter we will continue our pursuit of the theme of spiritual alignment through faith to the end of recognizing how God has provided practical help for us to receive the healing we need to be spiritually aligned with God.

The Spirit of God has repeatedly sent faithful messengers to us to teach us how to align ourselves spiritually with our God and Savior. Their voices "cry in the wilderness" of the many other voices that vie for our attention and loyalty, just as did the voice of John the Baptist as he prepared the way of the Lord. "God is most glorified in us when we are most satisfied in Him," these faithful expositors of God's truth proclaim.[1] This is also understood to be a message out of Jonathan Edwards' studies, which led him to conclude that we must "align ourselves with God in order to receive great joy."[2] C. S. Lewis wrote that being with God is like having an acceleration within one's heart. This meaningful acceleration is how Lewis defined *joy*.[3] And it is the greatest of all joys. Without this joy as the foundation of our lives, all other instances and experiences of purported joy evaporate into nothingness.

Paul wrote a beautiful book to the ancient French tribe in Galatia in which he declared:

> I have been crucified with Christ [in Him I have shared His crucifixion]; it is no longer I who live, but Christ (the Messiah) lives in me; and the life I now live in the body I live by faith in (by adherence to and reliance on and complete trust in) the Son of God, Who loved me and gave Himself up for me.
>
> —Galatians 2:20, ampc

The Galatians, like us, tended to become diverted by things other than Christ living in them. Paul was telling them that "now He is living in us by faith and by His grace. Let this be our focus before anything else." Later, in Galatians 5:1, the apostle gives us the great imperative of the book where, in essence, the Savior says, "Stand fast in the liberty whereby I have set you free. And do not be entrapped anymore." Here we see the true nature of our liberty. It is the liberty to love by faith.

This liberty to love by faith enables us to enjoy the fullness of God as it is described in Ephesians 3:16–19. There we hear the apostle's prayer for all of God's people. In effect, he says, "May you come to know God by faith, and may that faith be rooted and grounded in love. May you be granted, by God's glorious riches, to be strengthened by His Spirit in the inner person. May you live close to Jesus and experience His immeasurable and incomprehensible love. And may you be filled with all the fullness of God." His words are expressing the availability of the power of God living in you to make you stronger.

When you become stronger and filled with God's fullness, you are healed from the negative forces of fear, unbelief, and destructive desires. In joy, liberty, and faith, your healing is meant to set you free to glorify God. He requires your cooperation to follow His direction for your mind, thinking, behavior, and lifestyle, and in your spirit—all in a controlled and inspired way. You must be brought into line, into understanding and appreciation of the wisdom of His creation, evident in all life. Once you have acknowledged the beauty and majesty in the Creator's design, which allowed sixty trillion cells and two hundred sophisticated tissue types to emerge from the genetic data of a single zygote to form your body, you will glorify the Creator. Only when you learn to appreciate more fully His intelligence, wisdom, and caring for mankind can you apprehend the purpose of life, which is anointed by God to give you strength and healing.

If you are focused on the Lord, you can avoid the huge impediment to fulfillment and satisfaction: fear. It may be surprising to you to learn that fear is mostly self-generated. The fact that some people are afraid of the dark while others love it shows that our fears are unreasonable. Though we may not understand many of our fears, we can learn to defeat them with faith in God and understanding of our anointed purpose in life. Your obsession with fear can be replaced with your focus upon God's anointed purpose for your life. I encourage you to cling to this promise of Jesus to overcome your fears: "My sheep hear My voice, and I know them, and they follow Me" (John 10:27). There are many solutions to your fears written in God's Word, which He gave to help you reach the wholeness He ordained for you.

OBSTACLES TO ALIGNMENT

Earlier we discussed the key to your inner healing in terms of alignment to the Lord and His godly principles, which include a "blessed" mindset. However, there are many obstacles you may experience that will try to hinder your divine alignment for wholeness in God. Unfortunately some of these obstacles are internal, self-induced, and very persistent. These obstacles have the capacity to damage your well-being, injure others, and prevent the healing and abundant life that Christ offers from coming to you. They separate you from the Creator and blind you to His plan for your present and your future. The list of these internal obstacles that function as self-deceptions is long and probably familiar: selfishness, self-pity, worry, fear, the need to control others, and various compulsions and obsessions. We addressed some of these destructive mindsets earlier. Let us look more deeply into their destructive influence over our lives in an effort to bring them to the light of God, where they will lose their power over us.

Pride

Pride is an enormous hindrance to attaining the "blessed" mindset of wholeness in God. The Bible has a lot to say about the destructive power of pride. One terrible result of pride is found in this biblical statement: "The wicked in his proud countenance does not seek God; God is in none of his thoughts" (Ps. 10:4). Simply stated, pride prevents us from receiving the love of God and the wholeness He has ordained for our lives.

Pride, more than anything else, blinds us to the intricacies of creation and God's special purpose for it. Our scotomas, or blind spots, hide from us the irreducible complexity, power, and divine wisdom in the design of the human body, psyche, and spirit, which originated with a single, tiny zygote. It is pride that has allowed a cold, indifferent theory of evolution to gain prominence and influence over generations of minds. It is pride, then, that prevents us from acknowledging the majesty of the Creator and from worshipping Him in awe and appreciation as He desires. So it is pride, more than anything else, that separates us from God's grace, His plan, and the meaning and purpose for our lives. It is pride, then, that separates us most ably from our healing.

The root of pride is selfishness and unwillingness, through

fear and arrogance, to surrender to God's sovereignty. Pride is sin that originates within the heart. For some it may spring from undue trust in mere human knowledge and natural abilities (1 Cor. 8:1). Others develop their scotomas through a sense of self-righteousness, independence, or the artificial stature generated by power and wealth.

Pride will deceive you—blind you—while leading you into struggles in our relationships, causing you to develop a spirit that criticizes and injures. Most significantly, though, pride causes you to reject the Creator and the reality of His Word. This mindset amounts to a refusal to see His handiwork in the marvels of nature and the miraculous design for life and health. Without worshipful recognition of God, the divine source of healing, how can we experience His healing?

Unbridled pride will never result in personal growth, learning, or healing. Pride can only leave you wallowing in shame, debasement, and destruction (Prov. 11:2; 16:18; 29:23). Only your heart, designed and constructed by the Creator to be the seat of your inner man, holds the capacity for genuine understanding, wisdom. Only your heart can allow entry to the Creator's plan for your life here and in eternity and give to you His capacity for divine love. Once you confront the pride in your heart and repent to God for it, you will be astonished at the healing you will experience personally as you begin to truly love your fellow man. How you respond to and love others is a very accurate reflection of your alignment to God.

A critical spirit

At one point in his life E. A. Seamands left his successful career as an engineer to become a missionary in India, extracting his wife from her refined surroundings in the United States and settling them in a developing country with a meager one-hundred-dollar-a-month income. The two of them embarked on a mission that lacked not only a piano or a car but even running water and indoor plumbing. Once in India, Mrs. Seamands complained loudly and incessantly. Surprisingly even colleagues suggested to him that he would do well to divorce her.

Mr. Seamands' patient response to this was, "I can divorce her as you suggest, but that would not be what the Lord would want me to do. Alternatively, I can separate myself from her and her complaining and continue living the way that I want to live. Or, I can constantly pray for her and be an intercessor for her rather than her accuser." He decided to become this intercessor—to assist his wife rather than destroy her.

Through this difficult period in their lives Mr. Seamands surmounted the challenges they faced and became stronger in His relationship with God as a result. As he constantly prayed for his wife, she also became stronger and more tolerant. Ultimately the family ministry flourished through this couple's lives and ministry there. Mr. Seamands' love for his wife and his effort to align himself with God's more demanding and higher way of interceding for her had overcome her critical attitudes and constant bickering.

It is too easy to succumb to the temptation of harboring a critical spirit. Therefore, it is important for you to properly face the complaints and criticisms of others. It is necessary to intercede for them rather than accuse them. Accusations lead nowhere—except to acrimony and conflict. The only possible results of bitter criticism are broken relationships, division, and pain; there is no healing alignment for wholeness to be found in giving place to criticism.

Criticism of another may seem to have a momentary purpose if it makes you feel smarter or superior, but real purpose is found in alignment with God's desire that you love, forgive, and appreciate other people. By doing that, you will find a truly anointed purpose to your life rather than a critical spirit that is an obstacle to wholeness. But learning to love, forgive, and appreciate others will require that you die to self, consecrating your life to become one with the Lord. Only as you learn to move beyond the obstacle of a critical spirit will you find healing for yourself, your loved ones, and humanity.

A spirit of envy

One of our most intense inner battles is the one against a spirit of envy. Few inner emotional states have the same potential to destroy and cause suffering to yourself and to those around you as that of envy. It can rob you of health and well-being. The final, brutal influence of envy can be seen in the example of the world's first family. God had smiled on Abel and his offering of a lamb but was displeased with Cain and his offering of vegetables. Cain, consumed by his jealousy and overcome with anger, killed his own brother.

> A stone is heavy, and the sand weighty; but a fool's wrath is heavier than them both. Wrath is cruel, and anger is outrageous; but who is able to stand before envy?
>
> —Proverbs 27:3–4, kjv

It is a simple task to prove the repercussions of wrath as a destroyer of hope and loving communication, but envy is an abyss, an overwhelming weight. *Envy* is a four-letter word that characterizes selfishness. It represents a desire to possess that which does not belong to you. Envy is insatiable, never to be satisfied until it has wrecked the person in the vain pursuit to possess. Once that destruction has been reached, of course, the object of desire is no longer worth possessing.

As Cain discovered the hard way, nothing is solved by giving in to envy rather than seeking alignment with God and His ways. (See Genesis chapter 4.) An envious heart is filled with anxiousness and tension demanding to be released, which results in physical illness, emotional extremes, impaired judgment, and the destruction of the peace and well-being of other people. Such a power obstacle removes all possibility from a person of the alignment necessary for healing. Envy consumes the energies of body, mind, and heart. The only possible outcome of unmitigated envy is illness, mental breakdown, and spiritual death. The only way out of envy's grip is in purposeful dedication to realignment with the Lord.

One great temptation for those who are ailing, ill, or in pain is giving in to envy of those who are enjoying their vitality and physical and mental freedom. This sad phenomenon is not unusual; however, it demonstrates that an important part of the healing process includes the eradication of negative emotions and imagining. Healing can occur only in the absence of envy. Healing is, therefore, in part the absence of envy.

THE GREAT PHYSICIAN

Our understanding of spiritual healing must include the diagnosis the great physician gives in Matthew 9. There we read that Jesus said to these sanctimonious Pharisees, "Those who are well have no need of a physician, but those who are sick.... I did not come to call the righteous, but sinners, to repentance" (Matt. 9:12–13). Jesus is telling them clearly that spiritual health involves the need of repentance. The Pharisees did not believe that they needed the ministrations of the great physician. They were incapable of experiencing healing of the soul because they did not think they needed the heavenly cure.

It is important to understand the context of the Pharisees' status of Jesus' day. Bound by an empty, outward conformity to religious rituals, these religious leaders were inflated with a sense of their own righteousness and moral standing in the community. However, their hearts were full of contradictions and evil. They suffered from excessive pride and a wrong attitude regarding a relationship with God. Jesus highlighted their hypocrisy when He claimed that they were intent on cleaning the outside of a cup while leaving the inside dirty. Yet they felt no need for inward cleansing and purity that Jesus came to give.

Repentance

Why did the Pharisees not see that they needed repentance? Do we? Each one of us has experienced guilt for wrongdoing. Do you, though, try to compensate for that guilt with external actions that you believe to be right and good as the Pharisees did with their religious rituals? Repentance involves turning from your sin to the Savior. You must turn to Him for forgiveness. You must turn to Him to satisfy you. You must turn to Him to renew you and to heal you. Every believer must do these things to experience Christ's dwelling within them. The Son of God must cleanse the dirty, murky waters of our souls. He sends the Spirit to make rivers of living water, which flow out of your innermost being (John 7:37–39). Ask Him to give you a new nature—a new heart. This is the resurrected life. Your healing begins when you turn to God with your whole heart. It is then that you find the healing of the great physician. "You will seek Me and find Me, when you search for Me with all your heart" (Jer. 29:13).

Repentance always includes a new obedience to God. The apostle Paul calls us to present all our members and faculties to be engaged in a life of holiness. (See Romans 6:19.) Peter reminds New Testament believers that what God said of old still applies to us: "Be holy, for I am holy" (1 Pet. 1:16). It is interesting to note that the English words *wholeness* and *holy* derive from the same root. In reference to God the word *holy* means worthy of whole devotion; in believers it speaks of being wholly devoted to God. The original biblical words for *holy* in both Hebrew and Greek mean set apart. They remind us that God is set apart above all His creation and set apart from sin. For believers it means to be set apart to God as your Lord and portion in life.

This is why the Bible teaches that true wholeness is found only in holiness. True happiness is found in holiness. Spiritual healing is found in holiness. God's ways appointed for us are designed to meet all our needs. Behind each command are the Father's love and wisdom. Therefore, to seek our spiritual healing will always mean a realignment with the Word of God—with God Himself!

Repentance is never separated from faith. Faith is the act of casting ourselves upon Jesus. He says, "Come to Me...and I will give you rest" (Matt. 11:28). Faith is acting upon that invitation. The writer of the Book of Hebrews described it as running to Him. Faith is receiving Him as the Bread of Life, our Savior, our Deliverer. All that we need is in Him.

God calls us to find our satisfaction in Him. Do you see your need of forgiveness? It is found through meditating on His suffering the penalty for your sin on the cross. "In Him we have redemption through His blood, the forgiveness of sins, according to the riches of His grace" (Eph. 1:7). Do you need a new heart? He is the One who pours down the Spirit from heaven to show you your need of a Savior.

Peter described this mighty work of salvation by the Son of God on the day of Pentecost when he declared, "Therefore being exalted to the right hand of God, and having received from the Father the promise of the Holy Spirit, He poured out this which you now see and hear" (Acts 2:33). Do you need spiritual healing? He is the One who gives the balm of Gilead (Jer. 8:22).

When God revealed His Son to us, He said, and still says, "This is My beloved Son, in whom I am well pleased" (Matt. 3:17). The question you must ask yourself is this: "Am I well pleased to make Jesus my all in all?" He promises to be all that we need to bring us to heaven's shore. By seeing your sin with an unobstructed eye and turning to the great physician, surrendering wholly to Him, you take your first steps to spiritual health and healing. You must be saved to be healed!

Salvation

The word translated "salvation" in the New Testament is derived from the Greek word *sozo*, defined variously as cure, make well, get well, and restore, as well as save. Salvation is our healing and health. Two aspects of salvation make it so.

The first crucial aspect of salvation is that it was accomplished on the cross and that we must receive it by faith. Salvation rests in the imputation of Christ's righteousness to our account. This justification means that God credits all who believe in Christ as their Savior from sin as righteous. This is possible because of Jesus' work on the cross. He bore the penalty due your sins, and He offered up His perfect life as a sacrifice so that you could receive the righteousness of His obedience. All of salvation is based on Christ's death because no one could be good enough to be saved by his or her own works. The Bible is quite emphatic on this foundational truth.

> ...being justified freely by His grace through the redemption that is in Christ Jesus.
>
> —Romans 3:24

> Therefore, having been justified by faith, we have peace with God through our Lord Jesus Christ.
>
> —Romans 5:1

> For He made Him who knew no sin to be sin for us, that we might become the righteousness of God in Him.
>
> —2 Corinthians 5:21

The second aspect of salvation is its outworking. We must receive salvation by faith in a way that transforms us to the core. Many profess to believe yet are not saved. True faith and salvation change us from one who is self-centered to one who is God-centered and others-centered. In obedience to God there must be a focusing on our caring and compassion for others as well as our passion for God. The two greatest commandments God gave are: love God with all your heart, and love your neighbor as yourself (Matt. 22:37–39).

Real belief in Christ that results in our salvation results in our living a life that cares for others as Christ did. Resting in His redemption, pursuing discipleship in following Him, and caring for others form a threefold cord of Christian strength.

Forgiveness first

Ultimate healing—physically, mentally, emotionally, spiritually—will not take place until you have released any remnant of unforgiveness harbored in your heart. Until you truly accept God's forgiveness and then pass that on by your forgiveness and acceptance in love of others, you cannot live to the fullest degree possible. Unforgiveness is one of the primary obstacles to your health, healing, and meaningful life. Living a life of forgiveness becomes one of the first exercises to accomplish for healing, renewal, and communion with the Creator.

R. T. Kendall's book *Total Forgiveness* provides the definitive description of the importance of forgiveness in order to enjoy a full and anointed life.[4] The example provided by the Genesis story of Joseph's suffering betrayal, imprisonment, and defamation demonstrates the strength and character that can be forged in a forgiving heart. Total forgiveness is a biblical principle that we must embrace. To be capable of it may at times seem impossible. Yet to forgive the assaults that we suffer at the hands of others is a necessity.

God admonishes us, "If you forgive men their trespasses, your heavenly Father will also forgive you. But if you do not forgive men their trespasses, neither will your Father forgive your trespasses" (Matt. 6:14–15). To live in alignment with God—to meet the Creator face to face—we must offer total forgiveness toward all those who have harmed or hurt us. We need to possess a disposition of joy and laughter that can help us overcome and possess a reconciled spirit, which is full of mercy toward others, just as God is merciful toward us.

Forgiveness is a major key to healing because bitterness corrupts and refuses the existence of a thankful heart. Outstanding grudges and grievances can only cause or facilitate anger, illness, and despondency. Depression and a festering vengefulness, results of harboring unforgiveness, will drag one into darkest despair. A spirit that is bound in such a manner cannot allow the Father to teach or the Holy Spirit to anoint. There is no healing, then, in a heart filled with the malice and ill will that arise out of unforgiveness.

There is, of course, an additional dimension to forgiveness in our healing. Receiving forgiveness for our own mistakes, for the wrongs that we have committed before God's eyes and at the expense of others, is as vital to spiritual healing as being able to forgive others their wrongs. Dr. James Avery, a hospice physician, points to the observation that those who are dying often have huge regrets that revolve around a lack of receiving forgiveness or forgiving. Unforgiveness is an immense spiritual weight, and there can be no healing until that weight is laid aside. Dr. Avery has a prescription for people who are struggling with unforgiveness during the process of dying, which he borrowed from another hospice physician, Ira Byock. The prescription is simply a list of five things to say to loved ones:

- Please forgive me.
- I forgive you.
- Thank you.
- I love you.
- Good-bye.[5]

Human nature is sinful. We must actively seek forgiveness from those we have hurt and, more, from God. Forgiveness is a necessary precondition to healing. The *noetic* of sin—which is the mental manifestation of sin—leads to depression and illness. Not only do these shadows prevent a process of healing, but they are the antithesis—the opposite—of any pathway to healing. The noetic of sin and its inner illnesses can only be eliminated by an appeal to God's grace.

After the honeymoon

Healing is a process rather than an event, so it is a continual journey into God, who transforms us and fills us with Himself. Changes begin after the new birth and must be ceaselessly nurtured. As a new believer—after the honeymoon—you will learn that there is much to do to grow into Christlikeness. There are many areas of the old life that you must relinquish to put on the new life. Just as health will deteriorate in middle age through neglect and harmful habits, spiritual healing and continued health require vigilance, diligence, and constant attention. Every day of your life you will have a desperate need of the heavenly physician. You also have a present and pressing need of the Spirit's anointing to renew and increase your spiritual health. That reality insists that we find ways to wait on God in prayer and in His Word to receive His grace continually.

We often have difficulty with the discipline this demands. If you struggle with being able to receive or embrace Him with your whole heart, it is simply because it is human nature for you to rest in your own resources rather than turn to God. By that human nature you suffer from blind spots, obstructions, unbelief, hardness of heart, pride, and the distraction of seeking your satisfaction in earthly pleasures. However, God has a way of humbling us to bring us to the place where we realize that have nothing else to hold on to but Him. It is painful to realize that illness and trials sometimes accomplish clarity in your life. It is encouraging to recognize that healing occurs when you turn wholeheartedly to God and rest in His redemption.

Many times it is in your trials and, yes, through illness that you may draw closer to Jesus. Joni Eareckson Tada's life is a glowing testimony to this painfully glorious reality. She has lived life confined to a wheelchair as a quadriplegic since a terrible diving accident in 1967. Though the radical changes in her life were painful to accept, in that initial bleakness Joni asked God to show her how to live. In the years since her accident Joni has accomplished much for God's glory and in seeing many others come to know God's salvation.

Joni is a painter, public speaker, author, disability advocate, columnist, and wife, as well as a beautiful, joyful person. It was through her immense challenges that Joni sought to live closer to her Savior within His plan for her. She knows that by putting one's trust in Christ, concerns of the body become a lower priority. As she writes, "Life is intricately and intimately linked with Jesus. In fact Jesus is life—He says so Himself. So when we look for life worth living, we must look for it not in happy or heartbreaking circumstances, health, or even relationships. Life is in Christ."[6]

During times of ease and abundance we tend to feel independent and look to our own resources and strength. When life becomes difficult, though, it presses us up against Jesus. In hard times, crises, brokenness, and suffering we learn to depend upon God and His plan. This is healing.

"'Is not My word like a fire?' says the Lord, 'and like a hammer that breaks the rock in pieces?'" (Jer. 23:29). God sends His Spirit and His Word to be a hammer and a fire to break down our obstructions to faith. The soul's malady is purged by these heavenly weapons. Yet God also draws us to Himself by the sweetness of His promises, wrapped in the Lord Jesus: "All the promises of God in Him are Yes, and in Him Amen, to the glory of God through us" (2 Cor. 1:20).

Once you have come to know the Savior, your challenge will be to continue to grow and maintain your spiritual health. You will experience many assaults to your well-being, and each is a test. Only by abiding in Jesus will you continue to bear spiritual fruit—and to live a healthy, fruitful life.

RESTING IN THE BOSOM OF THE TRINITY

To experience God's prescription for health and wholeness, you need to have the healing touch of each person of the Trinity upon your soul. The triune God—the Father, Son, and Holy Spirit—is Jehovah Rapha, "the Lord our healer." We must learn to rest in the healing bosom of the Trinity. That is the essence of our healing.

We often begin our relationship with the great physician by coming to the Son of God as our Savior, as the only One who can forgive us our sins. We realize that only His death on the cross can remove the penalty of our sins and grace us with the righteousness of God. To know this forgiveness is to extinguish the guilt that plagues us, as well as remove shame and a sense of rejection. We know that by being forgiven, we are cleansed and welcomed at the throne of God.

However, many people arrive at an understanding of God as our Father only after following Christ for some time. There may be things about your earthly parental upbringing that still cause you pain or skepticism. Perhaps your perception of *father* is not a positive one. But God's Word has made it very clear that each one of us still needs divine parenting from the hand of our heavenly Father throughout our lives. You were created in such a way that you have an inner longing for God the Father's acceptance and outpoured love. Even in the midst of illness and suffering, when you sense your limitations and disabilities, you can rejoice that the Father heart of God has purposed the trial that you need in order to grow in His grace and discover new depths of His love. He has promised to work everything for good to those who love Him (Rom. 8:28). He is God the Father Almighty, and His sovereignty teaches you to trust Him and to "fear not." You can cast all your cares on Him because you know that He cares for you (1 Pet. 5:7). No beloved child will feel more secure or encouraged than the believing, forgiven child of God who knows how to rest in the redemption of the Father heart of God.

The longer you live the Christian life in this world as it is, the more you will learn how much you need the Holy Spirit and how much your inner peace and healing depend on your learning to lean upon Him. The Christian is called to serve others. The Lord Jesus did not come to be served but to serve. It is laid out so plainly for us in Galatians 6:2: "Bear one another's burdens, and so fulfill the law of Christ." The same is found in Galatians 5:13, "Through love serve one another." The Holy Spirit guides you into all truth and leads you into caring service of others.

However, as you serve others, you will find that they do not always appreciate your efforts. There will be times when you feel rejected and need healing for the wounds that result from your efforts to serve, so that you do not become weary in well doing (Gal. 6:9). As you offer up your service to God alone as a sacrifice to please Him, you will be comforted by the Holy Spirit. You will be victorious as you learn to live your life to please God. He is your cheering audience of one. By living your life to please Him, He will show you how to serve others also.

In your service to others there will be times when you feel the pain of watching others persist in self-destructive behaviors, which destroy themselves or their families. You cannot change another person's heart if that person does not desire to change. The Holy Spirit is the power of God who, in answer to prayer, can change the heart of stone into one of flesh. He can turn the hardened heart and bring reconciliation when all your efforts have failed. As you learn to rest in dependence upon the Holy Spirit's intervention, you will be able to persevere in interceding for them despite any discouragement you may feel. The Holy Spirit brings healing to the dejected servant of God who feels as if he has expended himself in vain.

The Spirit also brings healing to your soul when you fall into spiritual decline and seem to be far from God in a dry desert. At times you may fear that you have left your first love and cannot seem to revive the freshness of your "springtime" communion with the Savior. The prophet Isaiah said that when the Spirit is poured out from on high, He turns the wilderness into a fruitful field (Isa. 32:15). He pours out upon the dry ground of the thirsty (Isa. 44:3). He revives us again so that we may rejoice in Him (Ps. 85:6). This spiritual healing is available to every true child of God who is grieved by his or her own backsliding heart and who is unsatisfied with superficial, shallow Christianity.

The healing work of the Holy Spirit in your inner man is the wonderful experiential side of salvation. As you learn to rest in His redemption, He becomes in you "a fountain of water springing up into everlasting life" (John 4:14). He becomes a river of water flowing through your innermost being (John 7:37–39). The Spirit of God fills you, revives you, and renews you. He anoints you with His own gracious presence to give you a lively faith that sees this life in light of eternity. You will learn to live a life marked for eternity in the present moment. Abiding in Christ is the first and foremost imperative in your life.

Your spiritual healing is also dependent upon your finding your anointed purpose in a God-centered and others-centered life. All human nature tends to be plagued with feelings of insignificance and uselessness. The antidote to these feelings is an awareness of God's anointed purpose for your life, which is conveyed to you by the blessed Spirit of God. To have an anointed purpose for life is one of the greatest rewards of life with God in the here and now.

Through your nature—the design of your heart, mind, and inner longing for communion with your Creator—you seek and are capable of receiving inner healing. God's twofold gift of spiritual healing—forgiveness and a new life—are found in union with Christ through the cross. A new heart, an anointed purpose, wholeness, and eternal life result.

DISCUSSION QUESTIONS

List any obstacles in your life that have prevented you from aligning with God's Rx for health and wholeness.

Pray a prayer of repentance right now, and ask God to help you remove those obstacles. Write anything you feel God is saying to you as you talk to Him in prayer.

Write a scripture that applies to your situation.

CHAPTER 9

GOD'S Rx FOR **YOUR NEW HEART**

When you have the life of God within you, which is achieved in your spiritual union with the Son of God, you will be able to say, like Paul, "I live; yet not I, but Christ liveth in me" (Gal. 2:20, KJV). In your consecration to Christ you become a partaker of the divine nature, according to the Scriptures: "His divine power has given to us all things that pertain to life and godliness, through the knowledge of Him who called us by glory and virtue, by which have been given to us exceedingly great and precious promises, that through these *you may be partakers of the divine nature*, having escaped the corruption that is in the world through lust" (2 Pet. 1:3–4).

That is a picture of the redeemed life of God in the soul of man—in your soul! This divine life is called the seed of God within us (1 John 3:9). This wonderful principle of new life is permanent and stable; it does not waver or wither. It is wrought in you by the Holy Spirit at the new birth (John 3:3). The spiritual signs of the regenerate soul contrast markedly with the natural life principle in which we previously walked outside of Christ's redemption.

SPIRITUAL VS. NATURAL

Natural life exists solely in the realm of the senses. The inclinations and tendencies that arise from the senses exist in a wide variety of expressions among humans. For example, some people have strong religious inclinations. They may take interest in religious things as a result of their education or because they have fond memories of their upbringing. Others may be drawn to religion by curiosity or through intellectual engagement. Some seek the approval and social commendation that may accompany a person who practices a "religious" life. And others are motivated by the respect they have for the qualities of genuine Christian character they have observed, such as virtue and moral justice, honesty and kindness to others.

These *natural* religious inclinations are not bad in themselves; rather, they simply cannot be confused with the *spiritual* reality of a redeemed person living in genuine heart relationship with God. The person who has surrendered his or her life to Christ becomes a partaker of the divine nature of God; the person's inner being begins to be filled with the genuine spiritual qualities that characterize the divine love of God. And these loving characteristics are reflected in every area of the person's life and relationships. Christ's divine life within us is based on faith in Him, which produces divine fruitfulness from four branches of God's tree of life: love for God, charity to men, purity, and humility. It is Christ who provides the pattern for this life of God in the soul of man. In Him we see all these divine qualities exemplified—expressed in their clearest, crystalline form.

The Lord Jesus demonstrated His love to God while He walked the earth in His constant devotion, prayer, and communion with Him. The fire of delight was never extinguished in Jesus, and He remained diligent to do His Father's will, even to death. Jesus shows us what true love to people is in His unbounded charity, patience with His enemies, and His ultimate self-sacrifice. Christ remained pure, never to fall out of alignment with His Father by seeking sinful pleasures. And regarding our redemption the Son of God taught, "Learn of me; for I am meek and lowly in heart" (Matt. 11:29, KJV). He demonstrated the reality of this meekness when He knelt to wash His disciples' feet after the Last Supper. (See John 13:4–5.)

When we discover the character of God, we discover that He is exactly who He claims to be. Our deep assurance of that is our faith, which gives rest to the soul, bringing every aspect of our person into alignment with Him, enabling the growth of the soul into a reflection of His love. This faith originates in looking at Jesus' death on the cross, His pardon for our sins, and His example of living in the love of God on earth.

The character of God will be seen in your life if you truly love God and express your love in prayer and worship. Adherence to His will follows our devotion as the true delight of our soul. Worship and service to God become delights to our new heart. Humbleness before God and others is expressed in this divine free-flowing, self-moving principle of life. Then love—God's divine nature expressed in our love for God and love for our fellow humans—is the summit and apex of our new life of resting in His redemption.

LOVE

There is an exchange of your heart's affections in love. In that exchange you are refreshed and enlivened by the joy God possesses and the delight He shows in you. God's love to you far exceeds the love you can offer Him, yet even the tears of repentance and its sorrows have a sacred sweetness to Him when you pour them out before your divine beloved. Once your soul finds its satisfaction in God, then you can live from the strength of that felicity, facing all life's challenges in the power of His love. In that sacred relationship you are renewed and healed.

Your love to others becomes an overflow of this intimate

relationship of love and delight in God. If you start at the wrong place and do not seek love and satisfaction in God first, you will experience perpetual frustration because no human being can bring about this divine satisfaction. When God Himself is your first love and chief portion, then you find overflowing joy and love within your heart and soul to channel to others, independent of their appreciation or lack of it toward you. This is the divine nature of which you have become a partaker!

This satisfying relationship with God is the fountain of refreshment for your spiritual life and the well from which you must draw your motives for living. When you know the nature and reality of your new life and how to nourish and revive it in love, you will know how to perpetually find restoration and wholeness. You have entered into your realignment with God as He intended for you to enjoy. This is the health of the soul!

The essence of being healed spiritually and living life anew is found in your retreat from loving self and your abandonment toward loving God. Divine love is your delight in God Himself, beyond His gifts that He lavishes on His children. Every one of us desires forgiveness and an escape from hell to heaven. But even heaven without Jesus would not be redemption for our souls.

God's love within us is not a deed we do. Love is a reflex of the newly born heart responding to the beauty of God in Christ. A deed of love can be imitated, but a reflex of the heart's devotion cannot be. Love arises from the innermost part of the heart to revel in the beauty of God in Christ. To truly love God, we must delight in an intimate relationship with God that satisfies our hearts completely.

Loving God is delighting in, cherishing, savoring, treasuring, revering, and admiring God Himself, beyond any gift He gives—life and health notwithstanding. When we truly love God with all our hearts, independent of our requests and expectations, above our own needs, then we will find satisfaction, meaning, and purpose in life. That is the realignment Jesus came to restore to us through His death on the cross and His resurrection. Only in receiving His forgiveness for our sin—the cause of all our misalignment—is this love relationship with God made possible.

Loving God puts our hearts into a state of awe, contentment, and tranquility personified in our relationship with Him. This intimate placement of our person next to Him is resting in the bosom of the Trinity. It is resting in His redemption. It is to have Him in such a profound heart relationship that we do not need anything else. That is God's Rx for your new heart.

THE PURPOSE OF OUR LIVES AND ETERNITY

The inner healing found through the redeemed life—the life of God in one's soul—is ultimately expressed in an anointed purpose realized in our lives on earth. There is the deepest richness associated with an anointed purpose in your life because it has an impact not only for now but for eternity.

The meaning of the anointed life can be seen in the life of King David in the Old Testament. David was anointed by God because of his devotion to Him. In his youth he had made nearness to God his primary goal in life. He is called the "sweet psalmist of Israel," as he sang his devotion to God when just a shepherd boy. When Israel was challenged by the enemy, Goliath, and his nation, David declared his loyalty to God and defeated that giant single-handedly through his faith in God. As a result of David's devotion to God he became the greatest king of Israel. And though he was not perfect, he understood how to humbly bow in repentance before his God when he sinned.

The anointed life means asking God to anoint everything you do rather than attempting to live by your own strength. This abandonment to God leads to an epiphany of your purpose. The anointed life is, in essence, being a real Christian rather than superficially practicing a religion. This eternal significance of and meaning in life, this divine love in life, is only found when you ask for God's anointing—His Rx for realignment—and receive that anointing in Christ. Then life has real purpose—eternal purpose.

The anointing of that divine purpose makes your life in the present more meaningful, more productive, and more passionate. You develop as a godly person and accomplish to a far greater degree what would have been possible from your own natural strength alone, no matter your good intentions.

The Scriptures declare this beautiful eternal significance to this anointed purpose of life. This is the reward of a godly life. Scripture confirms it.

> But without faith it is impossible to please Him, for he who comes to God must believe that He is, and that He is a rewarder of those who diligently seek Him.
>
> —Hebrews 11:6

> And behold, I am coming quickly, and My reward is with Me, to give to every one according to his work.
>
> —Revelation 22:12

Your responsibility for this spiritual realignment through God's Rx is huge: your mindset now will be your mindset in eternity. Where are you focused? Do you sense your life has a purpose? Is your life meaningful? Will it be? It all begins with Jesus' call to you in Matthew 11:28: "Come to Me, all you who labor and are heavy laden, and I will give you rest."

The anointed purpose of life in Christ gives meaning now and for eternity. Everything you do in life will be judged by the Lord when you stand before Him in glory. Not only does He enable you to live faithfully for Him here on earth, but He will reward you in heaven for doing so. His Word clearly describes the path of life that brings blessing and reward: "You will show me the path of life; in Your presence is fullness of joy; at Your right hand are pleasures forevermore" (Ps. 16:11). Spiritual blindness keeps us from perceiving His best for us. The Holy Spirit is yours, as a believer reconciled to Christ, and He reveals the otherwise hidden diamonds of divine truth as you prayerfully search the Scriptures for understanding. All the criteria for blessing and reward are present in God's Word.

Those who reject the Lord in this life will be judged and receive eternal judgment according to that life here on earth. Those who have received Jesus as their Lord and Savior will also be judged for every thought, word, deed, and action done here on earth. In the New Testament, Paul understood this judgment and pleaded with the church to view life from an eternal perspective. The believers who had spiritual blind spots often missed Paul's challenge, as had the disciples when Jesus preached the Sermon on the Mount, recorded in Matthew.

Paul, well aware of God's grace, knew what it meant to be brought before a political court of law and judged for one's actions. In the Greek city of Corinth his enemies dragged him into court for preaching the gospel. Scholars believe that a raised marble platform, still visible today in the ruins of Corinth, was the place where Paul's case was tried. The platform was referred to as the *bema*, which is the Greek word for judgment seat. The *bema* represented authority, justice, and reward. Later Paul sent a letter to the church in Corinth and spoke of another *bema*—this one located in heaven—the judgment seat for Christians and the great white throne for nonbelievers.

As a Christian you will be evaluated by how you behaved during your time here on earth and rewarded accordingly. Spiritual insight for the believer, your inner health, is achieved by an eternal desire to live today with eternity's values in view. And God's eternal reward system is extravagant! (See Matthew 11:21–22; 16:27; 23:14; Luke 6:23; John 5:22; 2 Corinthians 5:10; Revelation 20:11, 15.)

Where you spend eternity is determined by where you place

your faith—in your natural strength or in Christ. The scripture declares: "Believe on the Lord Jesus Christ, and you will be saved" (Acts 16:31).

How you spend eternity is determined by your faithfulness. Matthew 25:23 says, "Well done, good and faithful servant! You have been faithful with a few things; I will put you in charge of many things. Come and share your master's happiness!" (NIV).

To be anointed by God is to receive meaning, direction, and purpose that God appoints, prepares, superintends, and revives along your journey through life. It is the interpenetration of God's Spirit and yours. You are thus divinely equipped so that you are not left to yourself. You are infiltrated with the Most High, with whom nothing is impossible. Anointing is God saying, "I have chosen you, and I am going to be with you!" Our spiritual realignment with God—our healing and physical health and wholeness—derive from the harmony, joy, completeness, and anointed purpose that spring from relationship with God alone.

TWO PENETRATING SPIRITUAL INSIGHTS

The Savior reveals many penetrating insights into the profound center of life, which are recorded in the four Gospels. They refer to true satisfaction and the nature of the divine healing of which we all stand in need. Two of these insights provide a special focus on the issue of our inner healing.

The first insight concerns what Jesus said was the one thing that was necessary—namely to sit at His feet and to feed on His Word and His person. (See Luke 10:38–42.) While Martha bustled with the details of her hospitality for Jesus when He came to visit her home, her sister, Mary, sat at Jesus' feet and listened to His Word.

"Martha was distracted with much serving, and she approached Him and said, 'Lord, do You not care that my sister has left me to serve alone? Therefore tell her to help me'" (v. 40). Jesus answered her with gentle admonishment, "Martha,

Martha, you are worried and troubled about many things. But one thing is needed, and Mary has chosen that good part, which will not be taken away from her" (vv. 41–42).

For you to receive all the good that the great physician has in store for you, you must choose "that good part." You must make it your focus to sit at Jesus' feet daily and learn from Him the joy of His fellowship, the wisdom of His design for your life, and His anointed purpose for your life. What do you feed your soul, God's Word or your own worries? The Son of God speaks very personally to each of us: "It is written, 'Man shall not live by bread alone, but by every word that proceeds from the mouth of God'" (Matt. 4:4). The question you must ask yourself each day is this: "Am I going to be a Mary today and sit at Jesus' feet, taking Him in, or a distracted and burdened Martha instead?"

Martha's actions in the account were founded on self-reliance and therefore were full of frustration. Mary's alternative of communion with her Lord and delighting in His presence represents a life full of satisfaction and contentment. In contrast to the busyness that Martha hoped would be generous to her guests, Mary's devotion to Jesus Himself generates a spirit permeated with the love of the Lord, which provides us the best preparation for serving others.

The second insight derived from a crucial passage in the Gospels is found in Matthew in the parable of the treasure hidden in the field (Matt. 13:44). Through that parable Jesus taught that our tendencies to pursue one thing after the other—in a ceaseless search for the satisfaction of our relentless desires—inevitably end in frustration and disappointment. In Jesus' allegory a certain man stumbled upon a treasure hidden in a field. Overcome with joy, *he sold all that he possessed* so that he could buy that field. Jesus is the treasure hidden in the field—we must choose Him with passion as the only thing worth having. We will count it a joy to abandon all else as the source of our meaning when we find our all in all in Him. As long as we have Him, we will be rich and full and satisfied. This must be healing, or nothing is!

Jesus is the Shepherd who will guide you to green pastures and beside still waters. He is the King who, by His power, transforms your disappointments in life into something good (Rom. 8:28). He is the heavenly Bridegroom who fills you with the love of heaven. He is the captain of your salvation who will lead you to be more than a conqueror. When He is yours, you can say, even in your weakest moments, that He is your strength. Jesus says to us, as He did to Paul: "My grace is sufficient for you, for My strength is made perfect in weakness" (2 Cor. 12:9). May you respond as the apostle did: "Therefore most gladly I will rather boast in my infirmities, that the power of Christ may rest upon me.…For when I am weak, then I am strong" (2 Cor. 12:9–10). This is why Paul could say, "By the grace of God I am what I am, and His grace toward me was not in vain; but I labored more abundantly than they all, yet not I, but the grace of God which was with me" (1 Cor. 15:10).

The grace of God enables you to fulfill the anointed purpose for your life. Even as you endure your experiences of illness and the breakdown of your health, He will show you how to allow Him to apply His Rx for your realignment to restore you to healing and health. Paul interpreted the disposition of spiritual vitality as "rejoice always, pray without ceasing, in everything give thanks" (1 Thess. 5:16–18). By living with such an attitude in life, you will receive the grace of God daily, which empowers you to enjoy the restoration of your soul's health. Truly resting in His redemption brings you peace, and peace is "perfect well-being, all necessary good, all spiritual prosperity, and freedom from fears and agitating passions and moral conflicts" (2 Pet. 1:2, AMPC). Anyone who can claim that peace as a reality in God is healed and restored to His eternal purpose for his or her life.

DISCUSSION QUESTIONS

What does *purpose* mean to you?

Do you feel you know what the purpose is for your life?

How does knowing God and His love change the purpose for your life and bring you a new level of wholeness?

CHAPTER 10

THE ROLE OF THE WORD IN GOD'S Rx

MANY PASSAGES OF Scripture that deal with healing and restoration point us to the power of God's Word to heal. This is encouraging because we have the Word of God in our hands and so can plead with God to fulfill His promises for healing in our lives by faith and the work of His Spirit. Solomon counsels us to cling to God's Word in our hearts (Prov. 3:1).

The mercy and truth that God speaks forth to you from the Word are designed to work in you a spiritual resolve that will "trust in the LORD with all your heart, and lean not on your own understanding; in all your ways acknowledge Him, and He shall direct your paths" (Prov. 3:5–6). God's truth embraced and lived by faith results in health: "It shall be health to thy navel, and marrow to thy bones" (Prov. 3:8, KJV). *The Message* paraphrases that promise like this: "Your body will glow with health, your very bones will vibrate with life!" The ways of God marked out for you in His Word are said to be "ways of pleasantness, and…peace. She is a tree of life to those who take hold of her, and happy are all who retain her" (Prov. 3:17–18).

Embracing the truth of God's Word activates in our lives all that is good, all that is honoring to God, and all that is concerned with true joy. That is how you find the satisfaction, contentment, and appreciation of God and His created gifts and joys. By doing so you implement the purpose God calls you to and you know the fulfillment of God's promises. You will know the joys of serving your wife or husband, family, and community (Ps. 112). By embracing God's truth, you will know the love of God poured out into your heart (Rom. 5:5). You will know how to deal with fear: "He will not be afraid of evil tidings; His heart is steadfast, trusting in the Lord" (Ps. 112:7; see also Ps. 91:3–7). You will know how to trust in God at all times and pour your heart out to God rather than "worry yourself sick," as we say (Ps. 62:8). You know your need of renewal daily and how to be renewed: "Will You not revive us again, that Your people may rejoice in You?" (Ps. 85:6). You know the fountain of life that is found in "the law of the wise" (the Bible itself!) and in the fear of the Lord (Prov. 13:14; 14:27). These two passages in Proverbs teach us that God will attend you in your serious pursuit of His Word with what can only be called a "fountain of life." This devotional life results in a life renewed to enjoy daily the majesty of God in appreciation for all His gifts to us and callings that rest upon us in a life with anointed purpose.

Just as your physical body is perfectly integrated within itself by the Creator's design, your spiritual life is designed to be integrated into the lives of other believers. It is not healthy to live a solitary, isolated life. Proverbs 18:1 says, "A man who isolates himself seeks his own desire; he rages against all wise judgment." The believer who knows the healing power of God's Word applied by His Spirit to our lives is a person who has the qualities that make a good friend and so enjoys the healing blessings of friendships. "Ointment and perfume delight the heart, and the sweetness of a man's friend gives delight by hearty counsel" (Prov. 27:9). Happiness, biblically speaking, is being restored through the healing of the Word—embraced, applied, engaged, and lived out in the community of believers!

The divine healing that comes from the Word of God is

described beautifully in the Book of Nehemiah. The captives who returned from Babylon gathered to hear the Word of God read and explained. The effect of that day was to teach them that "the joy of the LORD is your strength" (Neh. 8:10). This message of the healing power of God's Word is found throughout the Bible. We have noted before the truth recorded there that "a merry heart does good, like medicine" (Prov. 17:22).

Jeremiah found his source of a merry heart also came from embracing God's Word. "Your words were found, and I ate them, and Your word was to me the joy and rejoicing of my heart; for I am called by Your name, O LORD God of hosts" (Jer. 15:16). God's Word was the "medicine" he needed as he faced the difficult trials of the coming Babylonian invasion and destruction of Jerusalem. He knew the reality of God's intervention in his time of extremity, which is described in Psalm 107:20: "He [God] sent His word and *healed them*" (emphasis added). God sends His Word to us! We are often jarred off-center when illness comes our way; we easily get discouraged and flounder in a disoriented perspective of our lives.

The downcast disciples on the road to Emmaus from Jerusalem after the crucifixion of Jesus found renewed healing through the Word of God. The risen Jesus Himself came near to them and did not allow them to recognize Him. He asked them why they were sad and "expounded to them in all the Scriptures the things concerning Himself" (Luke 24:27). They later recognized that it was Jesus Himself who had come alongside them to reorient them—realign them—to God's Word. As they reflected on this experience, they summarized it in this way: "Did not our heart burn within us while He talked with us on the road, and while He opened the Scriptures to us?" (v. 32). God used His Word to stir the fire of faith in them again. In other words, "He sent His word and healed them" (Ps. 107:20)!

As with these disheartened disciples, who were soul-sick from grief over Jesus' death, in your times of illness you need to sense God's consoling presence anew. You need to be made functional again and hopeful and useful to the Master. It is the power of God at work in your soul that brings healing to the "illness" side of your disease. Your mind, emotions, and heart need the counteractions of faith and hope to renew afresh in you the "health to our navel and marrow to our bones" that He has promised you. Your hands, which hang down, are lifted anew in praise, and your feet, which are prone to stumble on rocky roads and be injured, are now put on the solid road to God's design for healing. "Therefore strengthen the hands which hang down, and the feeble knees, and make straight paths for your feet, so that what is lame may not be dislocated, but rather be healed" (Heb. 12:12–13).

How we need to be healed from our backslides of doubting God's goodness and despairing of His wisdom and sovereignty! Hosea calls us to this reengagement toward the living God: "In You the fatherless finds mercy. I will heal their backsliding, I will love them freely" (Hos. 14:3–4). When your expectations of health and usefulness are set aside by illness, you may say with Solomon, "Hope deferred makes the heart sick."

But he goes on to say, "But when the desire comes, it is a tree of life" (Prov. 13:12). We have all known the heart sickness of disappointed goals from illness, but now, with the powerful truths we have learned in God's design for healing, let us look to God to send the healing of His Word to our lives when we face each illness. He will be glorified, and we will be blessed. Then we will find our newly sanctified desires fulfilled as He has promised.

> Delight yourself also in the Lord, and He shall give you the desires of your heart.
>
> —Psalm 37:4

Prayer is the opposite of self-reliance. Joy is the opposite of self-pity. A thankful spirit is the opposite of cynicism. These negative dispositions are the things that destroy you; joy, prayer, and gratitude are the graces that enliven you and keep you living in the presence of God, who is your only source of lasting and satisfying peace. When this new principle dwells in you, you see the folly and vanity of life and understand that everything is contingent upon divine goodness and grace. When your heart is infused with God's life, you observe a wholeness and balance and understand that the love and joy you experience today, and the appreciation you can offer in worship now, are elements in your eternal life with Him.

Our benediction toward those who are seeking God's healing touch should be:

> *Let the anointing of Christ be in you, and His grace be in you, and the love of the anointed Christ who lives in you give you peace. Amen.*

The essence of God's Rx for your healing and wholeness becomes a reality for you in your abandonment to the Savior and in receiving all He is for your life—eternally—in cultivating a devotional life that will result in your resting in His redemption daily. As you become realigned to His purpose for you from creation and in His redemption plan for you in Christ, you will be able to pray these beautiful words of the psalmist:

"I will praise You, for I am fearfully and wonderfully made; marvelous are Your works, and that my soul knows very well. My frame was not hidden from You, when I was made in secret, and skillfully wrought in the lowest parts of the earth. Your eyes saw my substance, being yet unformed. And in Your book they all were written, the days fashioned for me, when as yet there were none of them. How precious also are Your thoughts to me, O God! How great is the sum of them!...Search me, O God, and know my heart; try me, and know my anxieties; and see if there is any wicked way in me, and lead me in the way everlasting" (Ps. 139:14–17, 23–24). Amen.

DISCUSSION QUESTIONS

How often do you pray and read God's Word?

What steps will you take to make time to do this every day?

What are the physical and mental changes you anticipate as you make this part of your daily life?

NOTES

CHAPTER 2

1. Edmund D. Pellegrino and David C. Thomasma, *Helping and Healing: Religious Commitment in Health Care* (Washington, DC: Georgetown University Press, 1997), 20.
2. Daniel E. Fountain, *God, Medicine & Miracles: The Spiritual Factor in Healing* (Wheaton, IL: Harold Shaw Publishers, 1999), 39.

CHAPTER 3

1. Ravi Zacharias, *Recapture the Wonder* (Nashville: Thomas Nelson, 2003), xv.

CHAPTER 4

1. "Clinical Trial Results Suggest Recombinant DNA Gene Therapy is a Safe and Effective Treatment for Patients With 'Inoperable' Heart Disease," Society of Thoracic Surgeons, accessed February 15, 2019, https://web.archive.org/web/20030624035521/www.ctsnet.org/doc/3148.
2. Pellegrino and Thomasma, *Helping and Healing*, 88.
3. S. Kay Toombs, *Handbook of Phenomenology and Medicine* (Dordrecht, The Netherlands: Kluwer Academic Publishers, 2001), 123.
4. Toombs, *Handbook of Phenomenology and Medicine*, 117.

CHAPTER 5

1. Charles Lasley, *120 Years of Longevity* (self-published, 2000).
2. Richard Steiner, "An Ounce of Prevention," Pro Health International, accessed February 15, 2019, https://

web.archive.org/web/20030410083532/www.geocities.com/b_sherback/matol_update7.htm.

3. Quoted in "In Case of Fire," Independence Hall Association, accessed February 15, 2019, http://www.ushistory.org/franklin/philadelphia/fire.htm.
4. Terry Dorian, *Total Health and Restoration* (Lake Mary, FL: Siloam, 2002), 137.
5. Ted Broer, *Maximum Energy* (Lake Mary, FL: Siloam, 2006), 14.
6. Broer, *Maximum Energy*, 14.

CHAPTER 6

1. See, for example: Chris Woolston, "Illness: The Mind-Body Connection," *Lifestyle and Wellness*, updated March 6, 2003, https://web.archive.org/web/20030802180339/http://blueprint.bluecrossmn.com/topic/depills; "Breast Cancer and Depression," *Artemis*, November 2000, www.hopkinsbreastcenter.org/artemis/200011/feature7.html; Chris Woolston, "Depression and Heart Disease," *Ills & Conditions*, updated March 26, 2003, https://web.archive.org/web/20030415213655/http://blueprint.bluecrossmn.com/topic/depheart.
2. "Mental Health: A Report of the Surgeon General," US Public Health Service, 1999, chapter 1, https://web.archive.org/web/20000303220041/www.surgeongeneral.gov/Library/MentalHealth/chapter1/sec1.html#mind_body.
3. William Collinge, "Mind/Body Medicine: The Dance of Soma and Psyche," HealthWorld Online, accessed February 15, 2019, http://www.healthy.net/Health/Article/Mind_Body_Medicine/1949.
4. Andrew B. Newberg, Eugene G. D'Aquili, and Vince Rause, *Why God Won't Go Away: Brain Science and the Biology of Belief* (New York: Ballantine Books, 2002).
5. James A. Avery, "The 'H' in Hospice Stands for Hope," *Today's Christian Doctor* (Summer 2003), 24–27.
6. Dutch Sheets, *Tell Your Heart to Beat Again* (Ventura, CA: Gospel Light, 2002), 20.

CHAPTER 7

1. Usha Lee McFarling, "Doctors Find Power of Faith Hard to Ignore," *The Tennessean*, December 23, 1998, www.tennessean.com/health/stories.98/trends1223.htm.
2. Studies include the following titles: "Religion and Blood Pressure," "Religious Attendance and Survival," and "Religion and Immune Function." See H. G. Koenig, et al., "The Relationship Between Religious Activities and Blood Pressure in Older Adults," *International Journal of Psychiatry in Medicine* 28 (1998): 189–213, https://web.archive.org/web/20031018090803/http://www.dukespiritualityandhealth.org/pastreports.html.
3. H. G. Koenig et al., "Does Religious Attendance Prolong Survival?," *Journal of Gerontology: Medical Sciences* 54A(7) (1999): M370–M376, https://web.archive.org/web/20031018090803/http://www.dukespiritualityandhealth.org/pastreports.html.
4. Randolph C. Byrd, "Positive Therapeutic Effects of Intercessory Prayer in a Coronary Care Unit Population," *Southern Medical Journal* 81 (1998): 826–829, http://www.godandscience.org/apologetics/smj.html.
5. Byrd, "Positive Therapeutic Effects of Intercessory Prayer in a Coronary Care Unit Population."
6. Byrd, "Positive Therapeutic Effects of Intercessory Prayer in a Coronary Care Unit Population."
7. Dale A. Matthews et al., "Effects of Intercessory Prayer on Patients With Rheumatoid Arthritis," *Southern Medical Journal* 93 (2003): 1177–1185.
8. Matthews et al., "Effects of Intercessory Prayer on Patients With Rheumatoid Arthritis."
9. William Standish Reed, *Surgery of the Soul: Healing the Whole Person* (Tampa, FL: Christian Medical Foundation, 1987), 53.
10. H. Helm, et al., "Effects of Private Religious Activity on Mortality of Elderly Disabled and Nondisabled Adults," *Journal of Gerontology (Medical Sciences)* 55A (2000): M400–M405.

11. Helm et al., "Effects of Private Religious Activity on Mortality of Elderly Disabled and Nondisabled Adults."
12. William S. Harris et al., "A Randomized, Controlled Trial of the Effects of Remote, Intercessory Prayer on Outcomes in Patients Admitted to the Coronary Care Unit," *Archives of Internal Medicine* 159, no. 19 (1999): 2273–2278, https://doi.org/10.1001/archinte.159.19.2273; "The Forgotten Factor: Faith," St. Joseph's Mercy of Macomb, accessed February 15, 2019, https://web.archive.org/web/20030218160513/http://www.stjoe-macomb.com/services/faith.shtml.
13. Larry Dossey, "Mind/Body Medicine: Prayer As a Healing Force," July 1996, http://www.healthy.net/Health/Article/Prayer_as_a_Healing_Force/743.
14. Dossey, "Mind/Body Medicine: Prayer As a Healing Force."
15. Harold G. Koenig, Michael E. McCullough, and David B. Larson, *Handbook of Religion and Health* (New York: Oxford University Press, 2001), 254–255.
16. See, for example, Linda K. George, "The Health-Promoting Effects of Social Bonds," accessed February 15, 2019, https://web.archive.org/web/20060504205318/http://www.cossa.org/linda%20george.pdf; Sophia P. Glezos, "Social Relationships, Connectedness, and Health: The Bonds That Heal," Summary of a Presentation by Lisa F. Berkman, Harvard School of Public Health, May 22, 1997, https://web.archive.org/web/20060502090712/http://obssr.od.nih.gov/Publications/SOCIAL.HTM.
17. N. Frasure-Smith and R. H. Prince, "The Ischemic Heart Disease Life Stress Monitoring Program: 18-Month Mortality Results," *Canadian Journal of Public Health* 11, no. S1 (May–June 1986): S46–20, https://www.researchgate.net/publication/19635319_The_Ischemic_Heart_Disease_Life_Stress_Monitoring_Program_18-Month_mortality_results.
18. Reported at "Depression and Cancer," McMan's Depression and Bipolar Web, accessed February 15, 2019, http://www.mcmanweb.com/article-43.htm.

CHAPTER 8

1. John Piper, *God's Passion for His Glory* (Wheaton, IL: Crossway Books, 1998), 47.
2. Piper, *God's Passion for His Glory*, 111.
3. See Earl Palmer, "The Christian Cure for Fatigue," Earl Palmer Ministries, 1996, http://www.earlpalmer.org/wp-content/uploads/2018/02/Fatigue.pdf.
4. R. T. Kendall, *Total Forgiveness* (Lake Mary, FL: Charisma House, 2002).
5. Mary Faulds, "Life for the Dying," *AFA Journal* (November–December 2009), https://afajournal.org/past-issues/2009/november-december/life-for-the-dying/.
6. Joni Eareckson Tada, *When Is It Right to Die?* (Grand Rapids, MI: Zondervan Publishing, 1992), 177.

ABOUT THE **AUTHOR**

James P. Gills, MD, received his medical degree from Duke University Medical Center in 1959. He served his ophthalmology residency at Wilmer Ophthalmological Institute of Johns Hopkins University from 1962 to 1965. Dr. Gills founded the St. Luke's Cataract and Laser Institute in Tarpon Springs, Florida, and has performed more cataract and lens implant surgeries than any other eye surgeon in the world. Since establishing his Florida practice in 1968, he has been firmly committed to embracing new technology and perfecting the latest cataract surgery techniques. In 1974, he became the first eye surgeon in the United States to dedicate his practice to cataract treatment through the use of intraocular lenses. Dr. Gills has been recognized in Florida and throughout the world for his professional accomplishments and personal commitment to helping others. He has been recognized by the readers of *Cataract & Refractive Surgery Today* as one of the top fifty cataract and refractive opinion leaders.

As a world-renowned ophthalmologist, Dr. Gills has received innumerable medical and educational awards and has been listed in *The Best Doctors in America*. As a clinical professor of ophthalmology at the University of South Florida, he was named one of the best ophthalmologists in America in 1996 by ophthalmic academic leaders nationwide. He has served on the board of directors of the American College of Eye Surgeons, the board of visitors at Duke University Medical Center, and the advisory board of Wilmer Ophthalmological Institute at Johns Hopkins University.

While Dr. Gills has many accomplishments and varied interests, his primary focus is to restore physical vision to patients and to bring spiritual enlightenment through his life. Guided by his strong and enduring faith in Jesus Christ, he seeks to encourage and comfort the patients who come to St. Luke's and to share his faith whenever possible. It was through sharing his insights with patients that he initially began writing on Christian topics. An avid student of the Bible for many years, he has authored numerous books on Christian living, with over nine million copies in print. With the exception of the Bible, Dr. Gills' books are perhaps the most widely requested books in the US prison system. They have been supplied to over two thousand prisons and jails, including every death row facility in the nation. In addition, Dr. Gills has published more than 195 medical articles and has authored or coauthored ten medical reference textbooks. Six of those books were best sellers at the American Academy of Ophthalmology annual meetings.

Did You Enjoy This Book?
We at Love Press would be pleased to hear from you if
God's Rx for Depression and Anxiety
has had an effect on your life or the lives of your loved ones.
Send your letters to:
Love Press
P.O. Box 1608
Tarpon Springs, FL 34688-1608